Principles of

Principles of Operative Surgery

Graeme J. Poston
FRCS FRCSEd
Consultant Surgeon
Royal Liverpool University Hospital

SECOND EDITION

CHURCHILL LIVINGSTONE
EDINBURGH LONDON NEW YORK PHILADELPHIA SYDNEY
TORONTO 1996

CHURCHILL LIVINGSTONE
A Medical Division of Harcourt Brace and Company Limited

◢◤ is a registered trademark of Harcourt Brace and
Company Limited

First edition © Longman Group Ltd 1987,
assigned to Pearson Professional Ltd 1995
This edition © Pearson Professional Ltd 1996
© Harcourt Brace and Company Limited 1998

First edition published as *Aids to Operative
Surgery* 1987
This edition published 1996
  Reprinted 1998
  Reprinted 1999

ISBN 0 443 050198

British Library Cataloguing in Publication Data
A catalogue record for this book is available from
the British Library.

Library of Congress in Publication Data
A catalog record for this book is available from
the Library of Congress.

Medical knowledge is constantly changing. As new
information becomes available, changes in treatment,
procedures, equipment and the use of drugs become
necessary. The editors/authors/contributors and the
publishers have, as far as it is possible, taken care to
ensure that the information given in this text is accurate
and up to date. However, readers are strongly advised to
confirm that the information, especially with regard to
drug usage, complies with current legislation and
standards of practice.

Printed in China
EPC/03

Preface

This is not a textbook of operative surgery. Its aim is to aid in revising operative surgery to the level required for the MRCS/AFRCS examination in the United Kingdom, concentrating on those operations which are commonly asked about and general principles relating to more specialised procedures and operative problems. However, it should not be regarded as the definitive syllabus of operative surgery for the FRCS.

The anatomist Frank Stansfield described revising as 'learning something for the first time the week before the examination', and the key to exam success as 'constant repetition'. I hope that by adopting the latter in describing operations, it is possible to avoid the former. The layout of the book is topographical: general, vascular, head and neck, cardiothoracic, upper gastrointestinal, hepatobiliary, colorectal, urological, orthopaedic and trauma surgery. Each description follows the same style to reinforce exam technique.

Liverpool, 1995   G.J.P.

Acknowledgements

I claim no originality for this text; most of these operations are long established in the surgical repertoire. This book is a distillate of the views of others, in particular the surgeons for whom I have worked.

I wish to thank my wife June, for her unending patience in the many months of preparation. This book is dedicated to her.

Contents

Introduction

HOW TO USE THE BOOK

The layout of operations is constant throughout the book, and by following it, it will be possible for the reader to describe any operation from the removal of a sebaceous cyst to a major hepatic resection. There are often many ways of performing an operation, all of which are acceptable, but for simplicity, I have described only one way of performing each procedure. However, if you wish to describe another way of doing an operation then write it down using the 'skeleton' described below. There may be other operations you wish to include in your revision and I suggest that you adopt a similar pattern for these.

HOW TO ANSWER QUESTIONS IN OPERATIVE SURGERY

An operation commences with preoperative preparation and the description should continue sequentially with specific points about anaesthesia, incision, approach, procedure and difficulties encountered, closure, postoperative management and postoperative complications. Questions may be phrased in a vague manner and the examiner may be trying to set a trap for the candidate; one of this type is to be asked to describe an operation like meniscectomy. The candidate commences at the incision describing the operation beautifully and logically, only to be failed at the end for forgetting to say that he would examine the patient preoperatively and mark the side. On the other hand, candidates may be reluctant to exasperate a tired examiner at the end of a long day by commencing on a long, drawn out description; usually examiners will interject in such cases and point out where they want the description to commence. If you adopt a step by step answer it becomes difficult to fall into any pitfalls of procedure.

PREOPERATIVE PREPARATION

Examine the patient and obtain informed consent, explaining any unusual outcomes such as colostomy or complications such as facial nerve palsy in parotidectomy. Mark the site and if the operation is ever on a structure which is bilateral, *mark the side*.

Special investigations
Those investigations which are necessary for safe anaesthesia (including sickle testing) and those specific to the disease concerned or operation should be described, including the amount of blood to be cross-matched.

Special preparation
Describe all procedures necessary to improve the technique or safety of the operation such as bowel preparation in colorectal surgery.

Antibiotic prophylaxis and steroid cover
Is it warranted and if so which drug or combination of antibiotics are indicated for this type of surgery?

Deep vein thrombosis
Does this procedure carry an increased risk of DVT (such as pelvic surgery) or are there any of the risk factors associated with DVT (smoking, oral contraceptives, age, etc.)?

Tubes
Should the patient be catheterised, have a drip or a nasogastric tube passed for this operation?

PRE-INCISION

Anaesthesia
Specify the type of anaesthesia employed, noting relevant points regarding agents and endotracheal intubation.

Position
Describe the positioning of the patient on the table and type of table (X-ray, Lloyd Davis supports, etc.) which you would use.

Skin preparation
Specify the extent, type of antiseptics used and placing of towels.

Position of surgeon
Describe the positioning of the surgeon, his assistants and where you would expect the scrub nurse to stand, reinforcing the impression that you have actually taken part in this procedure.

Incision
Specify the incision to be employed and acceptable alternatives. Justify your choice.

THE PROCEDURE

The approach
Describe the approach, noting anatomical landmarks and use of tissue planes (the examiner may wish you to avoid this and will usually indicate if so).

The procedure
Assess the pathology and any associated problems, especially expected co-existent pathology. Describe how *you* would do the operation, which sutures *you* would use, which instruments *you* would use.

Recognised problems
Note any common problems with this procedure and the techniques which are employed to deal with them.

Closure
Always describe methods of haemostasis and discuss whether or not drains are necessary. Remember the swab and instrument check and describe the closure *you* would use.

POSTOPERATIVE MANAGEMENT

Timing
Specify timing of removal of sutures, drains, tubes and dressings.

Specific instructions
Give specific instructions on postoperative management and care to be given to junior medical staff and nursing staff.

Special investigations
Describe special investigations relevant to the procedure (e.g. haemoglobin and transfusion, histology, microbiology, radiology and biochemistry).

Recognised complications
Describe recognised complications specific to the procedure, early and late and general complications of major surgery (DVT and PE, chest infection, wound infection, abscess, septicaemia, acute retention of urine, ileus etc.).

General surgery

PRINCIPLES OF PREVENTION OF SURGICAL SEPSIS

The problem
1. Wound infection
2. Peritoneal infection
    a. Peritonitis
    b. Abscess
3. Pulmonary infection
4. Prosthesis infection
5. Septicaemia
6. Pseudomembranous colitis

Sources
1. Autogenous ⎱
2. Exogenous ⎰ Needs an innoculum of >10^5 bacteria

Factors
1. Virulence of organism and numbers/concentration of innoculum
2. Local
    a. Surgical technique
    b. Drainage
    c. Ischaemia
    d. Obesity
    e. Foreign material
    f. Gut surgery
3. General
    a. Age
    b. Immune status (including HIV status)
    c. Pathology, especially malignancy
    d. Steroids
    e. Diabetes
    f. Cytotoxic chemotherapy
    g. Jaundice
    h. Uraemia

4. Organism
   a. Aerobes ⎫ Virulence and pathogenicity
   b. Anaerobes ⎭

METHODS OF PREVENTION

Prevent innoculation
1. Aseptic technique
2. Theatre
   a. Minimise movements of personnel
   b. Air change with filter, laminar flow and positive pressure
3. Surgical technique, care of tissues, haemostasis, no spillage, antiseptics
4. Plastic drapes do not reduce wound infection
5. Bowel preparation (*see* Colorectal surgery, p.104)

Antiseptics
1. Alcohol (70% isopropyl)
   a. Bactericidal but evaporates and is short acting
   b. Avoid in wounds since neurotoxic
2. Dyes
   Proflavine, gentian violet—useful with Gram-positive cocci except *Staphylococcus* and no use in slough
3. Formaldehyde (noxythiolin)
   Releases 1% formaldehyde and is useful in peritoneal lavage
4. Halogens
   a. Hypochlorite (eusol, Miltons solution)
   b. Iodoforms (iodine in alcohol)
   c. Both bactericidal and sporicidal, including *Staphylococcus*. Limited by patient hypersensitivity
5. Phenols
   a. Hexachlorophane—of historic interest since introduced by Lister
   b. Problems—absorption may lead to neurotoxicity
   c. Staphylococcal resistance
6. Quaternary ammonium (cetrimide, chlorhexidine)
   a. Bactericidal, not sporicidal
   b. *Pseudomonas* can grow in it!
7. Silver sulphadiazine (flamazine)
   Will kill Pseudomonas and useful in burns

Antibiotics
1. Prophylactic uses
   a. Appendicectomy
   b. Colorectal surgery
   c. Upper gut and hepatobiliary surgery
   d. Orthopaedic prosthesis surgery

    e. Risk of endocarditis following rheumatic fever
    f. Arterial surgery
2. Disadvantages
    a. No compensation for poor surgery
    b. Masks signs of abscess
    c. Development of resistance; selection and emergence, drug tolerance and plasmid transmission
    d. Toxicity–specific organs, allergy and anaphylaxis, agranulocytosis, pyoderma gangrenosum, pseudomembranous colitis with overgrowth of *Clostridium difficile*
3. When using an antibiotic for a 'surgical' infection, always consider
    a. Is there pus to drain?
    b. Is lavage better?
    c. Is physiotherapy more appropriate?
4. Always culture organisms and obtain sensitivity
5. Choice of antibiotic depends on
    a. Suspected organism
    b. Route of administration
    c. Route of metabolism/excretion
    d. Patient tolerance
6. Antibiotic prophylaxis
    Use for the shortest possible time, therefore usually only two or three doses commencing with premedication or anaesthetic induction for up to 24 hours post surgery (if the course lasts longer than this then it should be considered a therapeutic procedure)
7. Specific cases
    a. Upper gut surgery
       • Emergency surgery (*see* Oversew of a perforated duodenal ulcer, p. 80)
       • Malignancy (*see* Gastectomy, p. 82)
       • Obstruction (*see* Laparotomy, p. 87)
       • Strangulation
       • Opening the bowel electively
    b. Hepatobiliary (*see* Cholecystectomy, p. 89)
       • >70 years old
       • Within 4 weeks of biliary infection
       • Jaundice
       • Malignancy
       • Bile duct surgery
    c. Appendicectomy (*see* p. 105)
    d. Small bowel
       • Obstruction (*see* Laparotomy, p. 87)
       • Strangulation
       • Crohn's disease
    e. All colorectal surgery (*see* p. 104)

f. Vascular surgery
  - Reconstruction using artificial materials (*see* Principles of elective vascular reconstruction, p. 157)
  - Amputation for ischaemia (*see* Below and above knee amputations, p. 170)
g. Cardiac surgery
  - Open heart surgery, especially with valve prostheses (*see* Principles of cardiac surgery, p. 58)
h. Thoracic surgery
  - Lung resection (*see* Pneumonectomy, p. 55)
i. Orthopaedic surgery for joint replacement (either systemic, topical irrigation or within cement) (*see* Total hip replacement, p. 192)

PRINCIPLES OF PREVENTION OF DEEP VEIN THROMBOSIS (DVT)

DVT

Incidence (including subclinical cases) by labelled fibrinogen studies
1. Major surgery, 40%
2. Cerebovascular accident/multiple injuries, 60%

Aetiology
Virchow's triad
1. Blood
   a. Increased viscosity
   b. Increased packed cell volume
2. Flow
   Stasis
3. Vessel wall
   a. Compression (operating table)
   b. Trauma

Risk groups
1. Female
2. >40 years old
3. Smokers
4. Obese
5. Oral contraceptive pill
6. Longer general anaesthetic
7. Type of surgery
   a. Pelvic surgery
   b. Hip surgery
8. Malignant disease
9. Major long bone fracture and pelvic fracture
10. Pelvic sepsis

PROPHYLAXIS OF DVT

Mechanical
Compression stocking
Pulsion pneumatic compression
Electrical calf muscle stimulation
Foot pedals
Ankle rests to elevate calves

Pharmacological
1. 'Mini dose' heparin, 5000 units subcutaneously twice daily from premedication to full mobilisation. Reduces the incidence of DVT from 40 to 10%.
2. Dextran 70; peroperative infusion for up to 2 days postoperation. Reduces platelet adhesiveness and the incidence of DVT from 40 to 20%
   (Direct clinical comparison of heparin and dextran 70 shows heparin to be significantly better)
3. Aspirin, not proven to reduce DVT
4. Problems
   a. All increase operative 'ooze' of blood
   b. Dextran interferes with blood cross-matching and can impair renal function

Postoperative care
1. Early mobilisation
2. Avoid calf compression and leg crossing
3. Improve hydration
4. Graduated compression stockings

DIAGNOSIS OF DVT

Clinical
1. Positive Homan's sign unreliable
2. Swollen painful calf and leg
3. Pulmonary embolism

Investigations
1. Doppler calf studies
2. Plethysmography
3. Venography
4. Isotope labelled fibrinogen/streptokinase

TREATMENT OF DVT

Anticoagulate
Fully heparinise immediately and continue for 10 days, checking thrombin time and fully warfarinise for 6 months, checking prothrombin time regularly

Streptokinase
Only if the thrombosis is very large, with imminent danger of embolism and never in the immediate postoperative period or with a history of peptic ulceration

Thrombectomy
If venogram suggests that it is not fixed

IVC plication or filter

PULMONARY EMBOLISM
1. Associated with iliofemoral and pelvic DVTs, although only 30% have clinically proven DVTs
2. Accounts for 5% of hospital deaths
3. Usually occur 7–12 days post surgery

Effects
1. Minor
   a. Pleuritic chest pain
   b. Haemoptysis
   c. Pleural effusion on chest X-ray
   d. Atelectasis
2. Major
   a. Cardiopulmonary collapse
   b. Increased JVP
   c. Decreased cardiac output
   d. ECG changes
      • Lead 1-S wave
      • Lead 3-Q wave
      • T wave inversion
   e. Chest leads
      • Right side strain

Investigations
1. Chest X-ray
2. ECG
3. Baseline clotting screen prior to anticoagulation
4. Ventilation perfusion isotope lung scan
5. Pulmonary angiography
6. Increased LDH

Treatment
1. Medical
   a. Anticoagulate as for DVT
   b. Streptokinase
2. Surgery
   a. Caval interruption; plication/filter
   b. Trendelenberg pulmonary embolectomy

PRINCIPLES OF PREVENTION AND TREATMENT OF PULMONARY PROBLEMS DURING OPERATIONS

Patients at risk
1. Smokers
2. Obese
3. Elderly
4. Chronic obstructive airways disease
5. Acute infection of respiratory tract
6. Other pulmonary pathology (asthma, TB, carcinoma of bronchus)

Factors in airway narrowing
1. Reversible
   a. Secretion
   b. Wall thickening (partially reversible)
   c. Bronchospasm
2. Irreversible
   Airway collapse with loss of elasticity

Principles of preoperative management
1. Aims
   a. Identify risk and assess factors
   b. Minimise or eliminate effects of risk factors before, during and after surgery
2. Method
   a. History and examination
   b. Chest radiology
   c. Lung function tests
   d. Blood gases
3. Treatment
   a. Bronchodilators
   b. Systemic steroids
   c. Inhalation (steam, bronchodilators, steroids)
   d. Physiotherapy
   e. (Antibiotics)

SPECIFIC RESPIRATORY PROBLEMS

Arterial hypoxaemia
1. Especially in the elderly with postoperative confusion
2. Ventilation perfusion inadequacy with shunting

Atelectasis
1. Especially elderly and obese
2. Reduces tidal volume
3. Treat with physiotherapy

Gastric aspiration
1. Emergency surgery, especially for bowel obstruction (*see* Laparotomy, p. 87)
2. Haematemesis
3. Treat with steroids, antibiotics, physiotherapy and ventilation support

Pulmonary embolism (*see* p. 7)
1. Risk groups (*see* p. 7)
2. Anticoagulate
3. In severe cases
   a. Streptokinase
   b. Trendelenburg pulmonary embolectomy
   c. IVC plication/filter

Pleural effusion
1. Occurs in up to 60% of upper abdominal operations (often subclinically)
2. Increased risk
   a. Hypoalbuminaemia
   b. Subphrenic collections

Acute infection
1. Acute exacerbation of bronchitis
2. Bacterial pneumonia
3. Lung abscess
4. Empyema (*see* Drainage of empyema, p. 57)

PRINCIPLES OF SKIN GRAFTING

Skin grafts may either be
1. Free
2. Skin flaps
3. Pedicled
4. Free with microsurgical anastomosis

Free partial thickness (Thiersch)
1. Use on
   a. Large denuded areas
   b. Granulating wounds
   c. Site where contracture of the graft is of little cosmetic or functional consequence
2. Advantage
   Takes easily
3. Disadvantage
   Contractures which are inversely proportional to the thickness of the graft

Free full thickness (Wolfe)
1. Needs
   a. Strict asepsis
   b. Vascular recipient site
2. Advantage
   No contracture, therefore better cosmesis
3. Disadvantage
   a. No tolerance of sepsis
   b. Closure of donor site
4. No free graft will take on tendon,bone, joint surface or within a mucosal cavity

Factors in graft survival
1. Skin applied to healthy granulating surface
2. No subcutaneous fat transplanted
3. Accurate apposition to granulating surface
4. Immobilisation of graft
5. Revascularisation within 48 hours by capillary loops from granulation tissue
6. Absence of infection (especially haemolytic *Streptococcus*)
7. General health of patient

Graft failure due to
1. Failure of revascularisation
2. Haematoma/seroma
3. Poor immobilisation
4. Infection
5. Poor recipient bed (bone, cartilage, tendon, etc.)

Technique of grafting
1. Partial thickness using dermatome (free hand, power, drum)
2. Full thickness matching donor and recipient site and using scalpel to dissect out donor site

Skin flaps
1. Indications
   a. Poor recipient site
   b. Good cosmesis necessary
2. Specific sites
   a. Eye lid
   b. Cheek
   c. Intra-cavity
   d. Breast reconstruction
3. Types
   a. Cutaneous pattern flap
   b. Axial
   c. Musculocutaneous
   d. Free with microsurgical anastomosis
   e. Pedicled flap

4. Disadvantages of pedicled flaps
   a. May take several operations and months to move a flap from donor to recipient site
   b. Whereas free grafting performed at single operation
   c. May not match skin colour and hair

Free grafting with microsurgical anastomosis of vessels

1. Types of graft
   a. Cutaneous
   b. Myocutaneous
   c. Myo-osseocutaneous
   d. Osseocutaneous

2. Specific donor sites

Type	Vascular basis
Iliofemoral	Superficial circumflex iliac vessels
Radial forearm	Radial artery
Deltopectoral	Anterior division of internal mammary vessels
Scalp	Superficial temporal vessels
Thoracodorsal	Lateral thoracic vessels
Foot	Dorsalis pedis and long saphenous vein
Greater omentum (for surface cover or filling cavity)	Gastroepiploic vessels

3. Technique
   a. Anastomosis needs two patent veins for every artery
   b. Very accurate apposition with no tension and interrupted sutures using 9/0 prolene
   c. Very gentle tissue handling and meticulous dissection using jewellers instruments
   d. Full heparinisation of all vessels
   e. Nerve anastomoses – excise all neuromata and use perineural sutures (*see* Principles of management of nerve and tendon injury, p. 220)
   f. Use operating microscope unless the vessels are > 2–3 mm in size, then use an operating loupe (× 2–4 magnification)
   g. Problems – donor tissue is anaesthetic
      Graft failure due to
      • Poor vascularity
      • Sutures under tension
      • Vessel kinking
      • Extrinsic pressure on vessels
      • Haematoma

• Infection
If failure is suspected then inject fluorescein intravenously
and observe the graft under ultraviolet light for evidence of
fluorescence suggesting vascular viability.

INGUINAL HERNIA REPAIR

IN CHILDREN
1. More common in boys
2. Always indirect

Principles
1. Often bilateral (incidence of right:left is 2:1)
2. Often associated with abnormalities of descent (undescended
   and ectopic testis, see p. 151)
3. Often contains the ovary in girls under 2 years' old
4. High incidence of strangulation in the first few months of life
5. Operation at any age is now safe with modern anaesthesia

Preoperative management
1. Examine both sides and mark the appropriate side
2. If for strangulation, then sedate and place in gallows traction or
   over a pillow for one hour, if reduction then does not occur,
   proceed to surgery

Pre-incision
1. General anaesthesia with optional endotracheal intubation
2. Position – supine
3. Skin preparation of lower abdomen and groins

Incision
Groin skin crease incision above and parallel to medial inguinal
ligament

Procedure (inguinal herniotomy) (Fig. 1)
1. Divide superficial fascia
2. Ligate and divide the superficial epigastric vein
3. Locate the hernial sac at the external inguinal ring lying lateral
   to the cord/round ligament (the external ring overlies the deep
   ring in infancy)
4. In an older child it may be necessary to open the inguinal canal
   by dividing the external oblique aponeurosis lateral to the
   external ring to gain access to the sac
5. Very carefully dissect the covering layers of spermatic fascia
   and cremaster off the sac and gently separate the sac from the
   cord/round ligament
6. The hernial sac may be completely into the scrotum and

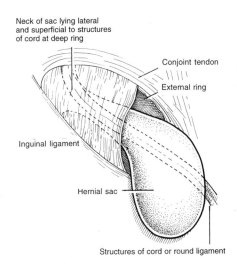

Neck of sac lying lateral
and superficial to structures
of cord at deep ring

Conjoint tendon

External ring

Inguinal ligament

Hernial sac

Structures of cord or round ligament

Fig. 1 Anatomy of indirect inguinal hernia.

therefore contain the testis; if so, then carefully divide the sac at the top of the scrotum and pick up its proximal margins in forceps; otherwise open the apex of the sac. In both cases examine and reduce its contents to the abdomen
7. In a strangulating hernia this should be done very gently as the mesentery of the small bowel and testicular vessels are easily damaged
8. Transfix and ligate the neck of the empty sac with an absorbable suture. Excise any redundant sac
9. Closure
   a. Close the external oblique aponeurosis if opened
   b. Close the superficial fascia as a separate layer
   c. Close the skin with a subcuticular absorbable suture

Postoperative management
1. Elective cases may be done as day-cases and sent home the same evening
2. Emergency cases – await the return of normal bowel function

Complications
1. Testicular infarction – due to cord compression in strangulated hernias
2. Recurrence – due to incomplete excision of the sac

IN ADULTS

Principles
1. More common in males (10:1 males:females)
2. 90% indirect, 10% direct
3. Operating for the second time in a male then it is wise to obtain consent for orchidectomy; such circumstances are usually exceptional
4. Exclude any predisposing factors
   a. Chronic obstructive airways disease
   b. Bladder outflow obstruction
5. Many operations and modifications have been described for this procedure, probably as testament to the fact that recurrence occurs with all, usually with an incidence of 5%.

Preoperative management
1. Examine both sides and mark the appropriate side
2. Chronic obstructive airways disease may well need preoperative chest physiotherapy (or consider local anaesthetic)
3. If strangulating, then needs resuscitation
   a. Cross-match 2 units of blood
   b. Broad spectrum and metronidazole antibiotic prophylaxis
   c. Nasogastric aspiration
   d. Catheterise

Pre-incision
1. General anaesthesia with or without endotracheal intubation (essential in strangulation) or local anaesthetic infiltration (60 ml of 0.5% Marcaine)
2. Position – supine
3. Skin preparation – groin (if obstructed, then prep whole of abdomen since a laparotomy may be necessary)

Incision
Groin incision 3 cm above and parallel to the medial two-thirds of the inguinal ligament

Procedure
1. Ligate and divide the superficial epigastric vein
2. Locate the spermatic cord/round ligament as it emerges at the external ring, divide the external oblique aponeurosis laterally from the external ring in the line of its fibres to expose the inguinal canal
3. Indirect hernia – lies in front of the cord
   a. Dissect the cremaster off the sac and dissect the sac and cord apart
   b. Open the apex of the sac, inspect and reduce the contents
   c. Transfix the sac at the deep ring and excise the redundant sac

4. Direct hernia – lies behind the cord in Hasselbach's triangle
   • Reduce the sac en-masse, unless large, then open, reduce
     the contents, transfix the neck and excise the redundant
     sac

Strangulating hernia
1. Almost always indirect
2. Open the sac and assess the viability of the contents
3. If the contents have reduced spontaneously to the abdomen, the
   constriction was probably minimal and they are probably viable;
   therefore manage as an indirect hernia. Examine the patient
   regularly postoperatively for evidence of obstruction or
   peritonitis suggestive of necrotic bowel warranting a
   laparotomy
4. If the contents look potentially viable, then gently dilate the neck
   (agent of strangulation), increase the patient's oxygenation and
   wrap the bowel in warm saline soaked packs and reassess its
   viability after 10 minutes. If viable then return to the abdomen
   (good colour, pulsatile mesenteric vessels). If it is not viable or
   is of doubtful viability, then resect the segment reconstituting
   the bowel with an end-to-end anastomosis

Herniorraphy
In all cases perform a herniorraphy to reinforce the posterior wall
of the inguinal canal. The guidelines of the Royal College of
Surgeons of England recommend either the Shouldice Repair or
the Lichtenstein Repair.
1. Shouldice Repair (named after the Shouldice Clinic in Toronto)
   a. If not already opened, divide transversalis fascia
   b. Using either steel wire or monofilament nylon, reconstitute
      transversalis fascia, and internal oblique/conjoint tendon in
      layers using a double breasting suture technique
2. Lichtenstein Repair (named after the Lichtenstein Clinic in Los
   Angeles) (Fig. 2)
   a. Close any direct defect using a non-absorbable suture
   b. Perform the herniorrhaphy by suturing a polypropylene
      mesh prosthesis in place using a non-absorbable suture
   c. The prosthesis must extend from the pubic tubercle to lateral
      to the deep ring, with its two tails extending above and
      below the deep ring, inferiorly it must be sutured to the
      length of the inguinal ligament and superiorly above the
      conjoint tendon

Closure
1. Repair the external oblique aponeurosis with an absorbable
   suture
2. For a repeat repair in which the tissues may ooze then it may be

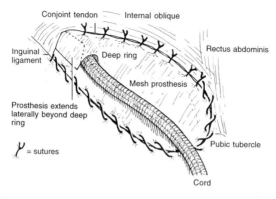

Fig. 2 Lichtenstein mesh repair.

wise to place a suction drain for 24 hours postoperatively
3. Close in layers

Postoperative management
1. Mobilise early; if young and fit may be done as day-case surgery
2. If strangulated, then commence oral fluids once the nasogastric aspirate is minimal and flatus has been passed per rectum

Complications
1. Hernia recurrence – 5%
2. Strangulated hernia
   a. Wound infection
   b. Anastomosis
      • Leakage
      • Stricture
   c. Ileus

FEMORAL HERNIA – LOW REPAIR

Principles
1. Extremely rare in children
2. Occurs more frequently in women than men, but even so, inguinal hernia is more common than femoral in women

Indications for surgery
All femoral hernias

Preoperative management
1. Examine both sides and mark the appropriate side

2. If strangulated
   a. Resuscitate and rehydrate
   b. Nasogastric aspiration
   c. Catheterise (empty the bladder as this may well be involved in the hernia)
   d. Cross-match 2 units of blood
   e. Broad spectrum and metronidazole antibiotic prophylaxis

Pre-incision
1. General anaesthesia and endotracheal intubation (possible to perform elective repair under local anaesthetic)
2. Position – supine
3. Skin preparation of groin and abdomen for laparotomy if necessary (*see* p. 87)

Incision
6 cm long over medial inguinal ligament

Procedure
1. Divide superficial fascia in the line of the incision
2. Identify the sac as it descends through the femoral canal medial to the femoral vein
3. Beware
   a. Femoral vein – laterally
   b. Long saphenous vein entering the femoral vein from its medial side 2 cm below the inguinal ligament
4. Open the apex of the sac, identify and reduce the contents
5. Transfix the neck of the sac and excise any redundant sac
6. Repair the femoral canal with three interrupted non-absorbable monofilament sutures from the pectineal ligament to the inguinal ligament

Strangulated hernia
1. Open the sac as for an elective hernia and send some of the fluid from the sac for microbiological examination
2. Inspect the contents
3. Gently digitally dilate the femoral canal (Hay–Groves manoeuvre of dividing the lacunar ligament with the rare risk of bleeding from an aberrant obturator artery is rarely necessary)
4. If possible gently draw down the strangulated contents of the sac, removing the agent of constriction and assess the contents. Increase the patient's oxygenation and wrap the bowel in warm saline soaked packs; if viable then return to the abdomen and repair the hernia
5. If the bowel is not viable but can be drawn down into the wound, then resect and repair with an end-to-end anastomosis. Return the bowel to the abdomen and repair the hernia

6. If it is not possible to deliver the bowel for resection, then perform a low laparotomy (midline or paramedian incision) and reduce the bowel gently from the inside. If the bowel is perforated then place soft bowel clamps on the proximal and distal bowel within the abdomen before performing the manoeuvre. If the bowel is not viable, then perform the resection and anastomosis via the abdominal incision (see Laparotomy for bowel obstruction, p. 87)
7. Repair the femoral hernia and close both wounds

Closure
1. Approximate the deep tissues with absorbable sutures
2. Close the skin
3. No drains

Postoperative management
1. As most of these patients are elderly, then day-case surgery may be impractical
2. Strangulated hernia – commence oral fluids once the nasogastric aspirate is minimal and flatus is passed per rectum

Complications
1. Recurrent hernia
2. Strangulated
   a. Wound infection (usually by organisms isolated from fluid in the sac)
   b. Ileus
   c. Anastomosis
      • Leakage
      • Stricture
   d. Perforation of bladder, especially if not catheterised
   e. Damage to femoral vein

INCISIONAL HERNIA

Preoperative management
1. Full assessment of aetiological factors, especially chronic obstructive airways disease which both exacerbates the hernia and may be severely embarrassed by the return of a large amount of gut to the abdomen by surgical repair (*see* Principles of prevention and treatment of pulmonary problems during operations, p. 10)
2. Would the patient cope better with an abdominal support and would the chances of successful repair improve with weight loss prior to surgery?

Upper abdominal hernia
Empty the stomach with a nasogastric tube

Pre-incision
1. General anaesthesia, endotracheal intubation and full muscle relaxation
2. Position – supine
3. Skin preparation of all abdomen
4. Incision – excise old scar

Procedure
1. Opening the peritoneum is a matter of personal preference and may be useful if combining the procedure with an intra-abdominal operation such as second look laparotomy in malignant disease
2. Freshen and expose the free edges of the muscle or aponeurotic layers for about 3 cm lateral to the defect
3. Close the defect with interrupted non-absorbable mattress sutures (Mayo repair) suturing one layer over the top of its counterpart)

Closure
1. A wound drain may be necessary if there is a significant ooze of blood from the tissues
2. Close the superficial tissues in as many layers as can be constituted

Postoperative management
Mobilise the patient as soon as possible; these patients are the same group who have a high incidence of DVTs and pulmonary problems, elderly and obese (see Principles of prevention and treatment of DVT and pulmonary problems during operations, p. 10)

Complications
1. Wound infection
2. Wound sinus from a non-absorbable suture
3. Respiratory embarrassment
4. Hernia recurrence

SIMPLE MASTECTOMY WITH AXILLARY SAMPLING

Preoperative management
Examine and mark the side; full psychological support and advice about available prostheses. Shave axilla

Investigations
1. Diagnosis with needle biopsy/aspiration cytology
2. Mammography/ultrasound
3. Isotope bone and liver scans for metastases and liver function tests for metastases are of little sensitivity unless the patient has very advanced disease

Pre-incision
1. Anaesthesia
   General anaesthesia with endotracheal intubation but possible under local anaesthetic if the patient is a poor anaesthetic risk
2. Position
   Supine with the arm extended and supported on an arm board
3. Skin preparation
   a. Avoid iodine if there is any risk of iodine allergy since a hypersensitivity reaction may delay postoperative radiotherapy
   b. Pack the axilla with cotton wool
   c. Towel up to expose breast and axilla on affected side with the arm towelled separately and therefore mobile

Incision
Elliptical at least 2 cm above and below nipple and including the site of the tumour. The medial apex at the midline and the lateral apex beyond the anterior axillary line

Procedure
1. Elevate the upper skin flap by sharp dissection in the plane of the superficial fascia, medially as far as the sternum and laterally into the axilla. Raise this flap as far as the clavicular head of pectoralis major
2. Elevate the lower skin flap as far as the inferior margin of breast tissue
3. In both of these manoeuvres dissection is aided by gentle counter traction on the breast and being careful to avoid button holing the skin
4. Commencing medially, dissect the breast tissue off the deep fascia of pectoralis major ligating the perforating branches of the internal mammary vessels
5. As this dissection proceeds laterally, beware
   a. Long thoracic nerve on serratus anterior
   b. Axillary vein above the tail of the breast
6. Remove the specimen for histological examination
7. Explore the axilla to remove palpable lymph nodes behind lateral border of pectoralis major for histological examination

Closure
1. Absolute haemostasis is essential
2. Place two suction drains, one medially and one laterally
3. Close skin in a single layer with interrupted sutures (a large defect may need a split skin graft)
4. Dress the wound with a support dressing for comfort

Postoperative management
1. Encourage early arm movement and test the function of the long thoracic nerve by assessing the ability of the patient to put her arm behind her head
2. Full psychological support and measure for a prosthesis prior to discharge
3. Remove the drains when dry and the sutures 1 week after surgery

Complications
1. Early
   a. Damage to long thoracic nerve
   b. Skin flap necrosis resulting in a defect which may need a split skin graft
   c. Psychological problems
2. Late
   a. Local recurrence
   b. Effects of radiotherapy (dermatitis, pneumonitis, lymphoedema of arm)
   c. Metastatic disease

ADRENAL SURGERY

Indications for unilateral adrenalectomy
1. Phaeochromocytoma
2. Cushing's syndrome, due to cortical adenoma (20%) or carcinoma (2%)
3. Conn's syndrome due to cortical adenoma

Indications for bilateral total or subtotal adrenalectomy
1. Bilateral adrenal tumour
2. Uncontrollable ACTH dependent Cushing's syndrome (78%) (pituitary or ectopic)
3. Advanced breast cancer (probably now redundant with the advent of steroid antagonist therapy: tamoxifen and aminoglutethimide)

Preoperative management
1. Adrenal localisation methods
   a. IVP – now superseded by modern methods
   b. Ultrasound
   c. Abdominal CT scanning
   d. MIBG scan for phaeochromocytoma
2. Preparation
   a. Phaeochromocytoma
      • α-Blockade with phenoxybenzamine (β-blockade only necessary if the patient develops a tachycardia)
      • Exclude multiple endocrine neoplasia (2 and 3)

  b. Cushing's syndrome
     • Large doses of corticosteroids from the time that the
       tumour or hyperplastic adrenal glands are removed
  c. Prophylactic antibiotics in Cushing's syndrome as the high
     circulating cortisol may diminish resistance to infection
  d. Control Cushing's induced hyperglycaemia during surgery
  e. Central venous line and pressure monitor
  f. Arterial pressure line
  g. Swan–Gantz pulmonary wedge pressure monitor is useful for
     phaeochromocytoma surgery
  h. Nasogastric tube
  i. Urinary catheter

Pre-incision
1. General anaesthesia, endotracheal tube and cardiac monitor
2. Position
   a. Bilateral approach – supine
   b. Unilateral approach – prone
3. Skin preparation of all of exposed abdomen and trunk

Incision
1. Bilateral adrenalectomy and phaeochromocytoma
   Extended midline or extended upper transverse
2. Unilateral adrenalectomy - paravertebral commencing 6 cm
   lateral to the spinous process of T10, descending to the 12th rib
   and following its line laterally to the posterior axillary line

Procedure
1. Anterior approach to the right adrenal
   a. Mobilise the right upper hemicolon and hepatic flexure
      medially
   b. Kocherise the duodenum
2. Anterior approach to the left adrenal
   a. Mobilise the left upper hemicolon and splenic flexure
      medially
   b. Divide the splenorenal ligament and medially mobilise the
      spleen with tail of pancreas
3. Posterior approach to the adrenal glands via the bed of the 12th
   rib which is excised
4. Beware opening the pleura (which may need to be closed over
   an underwater seal drainage system)
5. Specific points of adrenalectomy
   a. The adrenal gland is recognised by its golden yellow colour
      distinct from surrounding fat
   b. It receives at least three significant arterial supplies (the
      adrenal artery, the renal artery and phrenic artery)
   c. Left adrenal vein drains to the left renal vein
   d. Right adrenal vein is very short and wide and drains directly

into the inferior vena cava; therefore inadvertent avulsion can be catastrophic
6. Danger points of severe hypertension during adrenalectomy for phaeochromocytoma
   a. Induction of anaesthesia
   b. Lifting onto the operating table
   c. During handling of the adrenal gland
   d. Beware severe hypotension immediately after removal of the gland necessitating massive colloid transfusion

Postoperative management
1. Should be on an intensive care unit
2. Phaeochromocytoma
   Regular cardiovascular monitoring with colloid replacement for hypotension
3. Cushing's syndrome
   Replacement corticosteroids initially in large doses and then slowly reduced over 4–6 weeks after surgery (initially parenterally and then orally)
4. Commence oral fluids once nasogastric aspirate is minimal and flatus passed per rectum

Complications
1. Phaeochromocytoma
   a. Hypertensive crisis during surgery
   b. Hypotension after surgery
2. Cushing's syndrome – Addisonian crisis after surgery
3. Ileus
4. Wound infection
5. Late
   a. Phaeochromocytoma
      • Recurrent tumour in the other gland or sympathetic chain
      • Metastatic disease
   b. Cushing's
      • Hyperplasia of residual gland if resection is inadequate

LAPAROTOMY FOR PERITONITIS OF UNKNOWN CAUSE
Preoperative management
1. Resuscitation
   a. Intravenous fluids, especially colloids to restore the blood pressure
   b. Nasogastric aspiration
   c. Central venous pressure monitor
   d. Catheterise to monitor urine output
2. Investigation
   a. Full blood count and electrolyte estimation
   b. Blood for microbiological culture

   c. Erect abdominal X-ray
- Subphrenic gas
- Obstruction

   d. ECG – exclude myocardial infarction as a cause of the pain

   e. Chest X-ray – exclude lower lobe pneumonia as a cause of the pain

   f. Urine microscopy

   g. Amylase to exclude pancreatitis

3. Informed consent, warning of the possibility of a defunctioning colostomy if the peritonitis is due to colonic pathology
4. Broad spectrum antibiotics and metronidazole for a full therapeutic course

Pre-incision
1. General anaesthesia with endotracheal intubation
2. Position – supine
3. Skin preparation of all of abdomen (nipples to thighs)
4. Towel up to expose midline but able to extend incision to either xiphisternum or symphysis pubis

Incision
Periumbilical midline

Procedure
1. Pack off walls of wound with antiseptic soaked packs before opening the peritoneum
2. Upon opening the peritoneum aspirate any free pus. Swab with a bacteriological throat swab and send this specimen for gram staining, culture and sensitivity
3. Open the peritoneum for the length of the wound and suck out all the free fluid
4. Gently perform a laparotomy to ascertain the cause (the smell of the gas released is usually indicative of the site; high gastrointestinal causes are initially odourless whereas colonic perforation smells faeculent)
5. Perform appropriate surgery (see relevant section)

Closure
1. Prior to closure, mop out the peritoneal cavity, including all its recesses and spaces for solid infected debris
2. Gently irrigate the peritoneum with several litres of warm saline, continuously sucking this out to reduce the concentration of innoculating pathogenic organisms
3. Close in layers

Controversies of management
1. Intraperitoneal lavage with topical antibiotics and antiseptics (e.g. tetracycline)
   Wound drainage
   Antiseptic wound irrigation

Postoperative management
1. Continue parenteral antibiotics for a full therapeutic course
2. Commence oral fluids once the nasogastric aspirate is minimal and flatus is passed per rectum

Complications
1. Immediate
   a. Septicaemia
   b. Wound infection
   c. (Portal pyaemia)
2. First month
   a. Intraperitoneal abscess
   b. Obstruction
      • Ileus
      • Adhesions
      • Anastomotic oedema
3. Late
   a. Incisional hernia
   b. Obstruction
      • Adhesions
      • Anastomotic stricture

DRAINAGE OF AN INTRA-ABDOMINAL ABSCESS
Preoperative management
1. Establish the diagnosis
   a. Clinically, swinging pyrexia and malaise 1 week after abdominal surgery or trauma
   b. May be tender over the site of a collection
2. Investigations
   a. Leucocytosis
   b. Raised alkaline phosphatase
   c. Chest X-ray may show gas filled subphrenic loculus with a fluid level
   d. Ultrasound CT localisation – allows aspiration of pus to confirm the diagnosis with microbiological examination and percutaneous drainage
   e. Indium labelled leucocyte scan (not widely available)
3. Antibiotic prophylaxis (cephalosporin and metronidazole) to reduce the risk of septicaemia
4. Drainage is necessary as soon as the diagnosis is made

Pre-incision
1. General anaesthesia and endotracheal intubation
2. Position – supine, unless
    a. Posterior subphrenic – lateral position
    b. Pelvic abscess – lithotomy position
3. Skin preparation of whole of abdomen
4. Incision
    a. Over the site of the abscess
    b. Pelvic abscess, which is bulging into the anterior rectum; drain via the rectum

Procedure
1. The aim of drainage is to evacuate the pus, with minimal disturbance of the wall of the abscess in continuity with the peritoneum, therefore minimising intraperitoneal spillage
2. Send pus for microbiological examination
3. Gently digitally break down loculi
4. Appendix abscess – unless the appendix is obviously lying free within the abscess cavity and easily removable it should be left alone and removed electively 2–3 months later
5. Drainage – place a large tube drain into the cavity and bring out through a separate incision (except rectally drained pelvic abscesses where this is impractical)

Closure
1. Irrigate the wound with antiseptic
2. Close in layers with interrupted absorbable sutures
3. Secure the drain with a stout suture

Postoperative management
1. Continue parenteral antibiotics until apyrexial
2. Rectally drained pelvic abscess – needs daily rectal examination to prevent loculation of the cavity
3. When the drainage is minimal and serous then gradually shorten the drain allowing the cavity to collapse
4. If the drainage is persistent then consider a sinogram to exclude a fistula to the bowel
5. Culture any persistently purulent discharge

Complications
1. Early
    a. Septicaemia
    b. Fistula
    c. Wound infection
    d. Recurrent abscess
2. Late
    a. Fistula
    b. Recurrent abscess
    c. Incisional hernia

Head and neck surgery

SUPERFICIAL PAROTIDECTOMY

Preoperative management
Examine the patient and mark the side, explain risk to VIIth nerve and exclude any prior VIIth nerve weakness

Investigation
1. Group and save
2. Plain X-ray of parotid region
3. Sialogram (stone disease, may show tumour in deep lobe)
4. CT/MRI scan of parotid gland to show relationship of tumour to deep structures

Special preparation
Shave side of face to temple

Pre-incision
1. Anaesthesia
   a. General with endotracheal intubation
   b. Avoid long acting muscle relaxants as they render the nerve stimulator ineffectual especially when seeking the smaller divisions of the facial nerve
2. Position
   a. Supine with head supported and tilted slightly away from affected side
   b. A slight head up tilt on the table relieves venous congestion
3. Preparation
   a. Towel up with the whole of the face exposed, or drape the face in translucent plastic allowing assessment of stimulation of all branches of VIIth during dissection

Incision (Fig. 3)
Pre-auricular extending under ear and down anterior border of sternomastoid

29

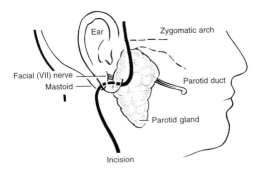

Fig. 3 Position of incision for superficial parotidectomy.

Procedure
1. Elevate the skin flap anteriorly with skin hooks and locate the origin of the VIIth nerve lying anterior to the mastoid process; inferior to the bony external auditory meatus, emerging from the stylo mastoid foramen and lateral to styloid process
   a. NB It lies 1 cm medio-inferiorly to the pointed end of the trigonal cartilage of the ear
   b. The trunk lies deep to the finger nail of an index finger placed with the distal interphalangeal joint on the mastoid process (Beahrs)
   c. The main trunk bisects an angle between posterior belly of digastric and the bony tympanic plate
   d. Its position can be elicited by use of a nerve stimulator, watching the effects of stimulation on the facial muscle groups (especially useful for the smaller divisions)
2. Locate and preserve greater auricular nerve for use if nerve grafting of the facial nerve is necessary
3. Since the VIIth nerve becomes very superficial anteriorly never elevate the anterior skin flap further than the dissection of the parotid gland
4. Dissect superficial parotid from deep parotid in the plane of the facial nerve
5. If the tumour involves the nerve then the central divisions may be sacrificed since they have good anastomoses, but superior and inferior division should be replaced by nerve graft if it is necessary to excise them
6. Structures to beware
   a. VIIth nerve
   b. Parotid duct
   c. External carotid artery and retromandibular vein deep to VIIth nerve

7. Remove the specimen after ligation and division of the parotid duct

Closure
1. Absolute haemostasis
2. Suction drain to wound
3. Oppose edges with several subcutaneous sutures and close skin with interrupted fine monofilament sutures

Post-operative management
Remove
   a. Drain when dry, 24 hours
   b. Sutures, 2–3 days

Investigations
Histology of specimen

Complications
1. VIIth nerve damage, usually neuropraxia. If permanent then consider
   a. Hypoglossal hitch
   b. Nerve graft with greater auricular nerve donor
   c. Plastic surgery
2. Fistula, usually closes spontaneously; if persists then treat with radiotherapy *Gustatory sweating*
3. Frey's syndrome, due to disorganisation of postganglionic sympathetic fibres and preganglionic parasympathetic fibres. Treatment: divide greater superficial petrosal nerve carrying preganglionic parasympathetic fibres (tympanic neurectomy)

4. Great Auricula Nerve damage

EXCISION OF SUBMANDIBULAR GLAND
Preoperative management
1. Examine and mark the side
2. Assess
   a. Hypoglossal nerve
   b. Mandibular branch of facial nerve
   c. Lingual nerve
3. Shave chin and neck

Special investigations
1. Sialogram
2. Plain X-rays of floor of mouth

Pre-incision
1. Anaesthesia
   General anaesthesia with endotracheal intubation
2. Position
   Supine, with head supported on a ring, extended on neck and turned away

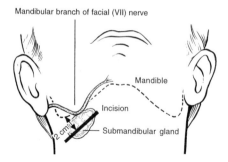

Fig. 4 Incision for excision at submandibular gland.

3. Skin preparation from mouth to lower neck with separate head towel
4. Expose face and lower mouth

Incision (Fig. 4)
Parallel and at least 2 cm below line of posterior third of mandible, thus avoiding mandibular branch of facial nerve

Procedure
1. Divide platysma and deep cervical fascia in the line of the incision to expose the lower pole of gland and dissect it free
2. Retract posteriorly
   Posterior belly of digastric and stylohyoid
3. Doubly ligate and divide the facial artery as it enters the posterior operative field
4. Retract meylohyoid, explosing the deep part of the gland
5. Dissect out the deep gland
6. Beware
   a. Hypoglossal nerve lying on hypoglossus deep to the gland
   b. Lingual nerve
7. Ligate and divide Wharton's duct – protect lingual nerve passing anteriorly underneath from lateral to medial
8. Remove gland

Closure
1. Meticulous haemostasis
2. Suction drain to wound
3. Close in layers

Postoperative management
Remove
1. Suction drain when dry
2. Sutures at 3–5 days

Special investigation
Histology of gland

Complications
1. Nerve damage
   a. Mandibular branch of VIIth nerve
   b. Hypoglossal nerve
   c. Lingual nerve
2. Infection
3. Submandibular fistula is very uncommon

EXCISION OF A STONE IN THE SUBMANDIBULAR DUCT

Indications
1. Impaction of a calculus at or near the orifice of the submandibular duct
2. Posterior duct stones should be treated by excision of the submandibular gland (see p. 31)

Preoperative management
1. Investigations
   Plain X-ray of the floor of the mouth
2. Broad spectrum antibiotics if concomittant submandibular sialoadenitis
3. IVI

Pre-incision
1. General anaesthesia with nasotracheal intubation and pharyngeal pack
2. Position
   a. Supine with head supported
   b. Mouth kept open with self retaining retractor

Procedure
1. Palpate the stone gently, avoid pushing it backwards into the gland. Impalpable stone: do not proceed
2. Retract the tongue to the opposite side
3. Pass a catgut suture under the duct behind the stone to prevent it slipping backwards
4. Pass a similar suture under the duct immediately in front of the stone
5. Beware passing the sutures too deeply as the lingual nerve is passing under duct
6. Incise the duct directly over the calculus and lift the stone out of the duct

Closure
1. Haemostasis
2. Do not close opening in duct
3. Remove pharyngeal pack

Postoperative management
Culture any pus exuding from duct

Complications
1. Early
   a. Sialoadenitis
   b. Reactionary haemorrhage
2. Late
   a. Recurrent stone
   b. Consider excision of submandibular gland (see p. 31)

TRACHEOSTOMY

Indications
1. Improve ventilation
2. Relieve obstructed airway
3. Radical head and neck surgery
4. Assist bronchial toilet, respiratory care

Preoperative management
1. Investigations
   a. Respiratory function tests – blood gases
   b. Chest X-ray
2. Shave neck
3. Antibiotics
   If indicated as a result of microbiological results from sputum
4. Endotracheal tube may already be in situ
5. IVI
6. Catheter/NG tube usually already in situ because of requirements for tracheostomy

Pre-incision
1. Anaesthesia, either
   a. Local (infiltrate 1% lignocaine with 1:300 000 adrenaline)
   b. General
2. Position supine, shoulders elevated on a sandbag with the neck extended
3. Check proposed tube – size and cuff function
4. Towel up, paint mouth to nipple with head towelled in separate head towel

Incision
1. Elective
   Transverse 2 cm above sternal notch – 5 cm long
2. Emergency
   a. Vertical immediately above sternal notch
   b. Consider crico-thyroid stab
3. Beware, in babies the innominate vein may lie above the sternal notch

Procedure
1. Deepen incision through platysma and deep cervical fascia
2. Open the strap muscle longitudinally in the midline
3. Divide the thyroid isthmus between haemostats and oversew the free edges with an absorbable suture to maintain haemostasis
4. If performed under local anaesthetic, inject trachea directly and spray mucosa with 2 ml of 1% lignocaine to depress the cough reflex
5. Open trachea (Fig. 5)
   a. Lift up cricoid cartilage with hook
   b. Cut out disc of 3rd ring 1 cm in width or create a Bjork flap based on the 4th tracheal ring
   c. Visualise endotracheal tube
6. Remove endotracheal tube, insert tracheostomy tube and obturator, remove obturator and attach the tracheostomy tube to the ventilator
7. Secure the tube with ties

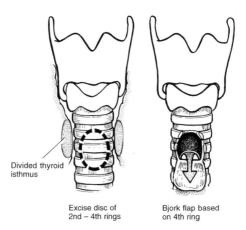

Divided thyroid
isthmus

Excise disc of   Bjork flap based
2nd – 4th rings   on 4th ring

Fig. 5 Methods of opening trachea at tracheostomy.

Closure
1. Absolute haemostasis
2. No drain
3. Close very loosely in layers around the tracheostomy tube

Postoperative management
1. Half-hourly observation until stable on intensive care unit
2. At bedside
   a. Humidifier
   b. Oxygen for tracheostomy tube
   c. Suction
   d. Dressing pack
   e. Retractor
   f. Tracheal dilator
   g. Good overhead light

Investigation
1. Chest X-ray
   a. Position of tube
   b. Exclude pneumothorax/surgical emphysema
2. Blood gases
3. Remove sutures, 5–7 days
4. If breathing spontaneously consider changing tube to a silver speaking type

Complications
1. Early
   a. Surgical emphysema, especially in the mediastinum
   b. Pneumothorax
   c. Tube
      • Obstruction
      • Displacement
   d. Tracheal/tube encrustation
   e. Haemorrhage
      • Reactionary
      • Secondary
2. Late
   a. Tracheal stenosis
   b. Trachea-cutaneous fistula

SUBTOTAL THYROIDECTOMY

Preoperative management
1. Warn patient of the incidence of postoperative hypothyroidism and recurrent hyperthyroidism in Graves' disease
2. Special investigations
   a. Thyroid

- Thyroid function test and antibodies
- Isotope uptake scans
- Plasma calcium level
- Indirect laryngoscopy to check cords
b. Blood group and save
3. Special preparation
   a. If hyperthyroid then render as euthyroid as possible preoperatively with carbimazole and propranolol and continue propranolol for at least 10 days postoperatively
   b. Lugol's iodine for 2 weeks preoperatively reduces the vascularity of the gland
4. IVI

Pre-incision
1. Anaesthesia – general anaesthesia with endotracheal intubation
2. Position supine with shoulders supported on a sandbag and neck extended
   Support head on a ring. 5° head up tilt of operating table reduces venous engorgement
3. Surgeon on side opposite lobe to be operated upon
4. Skin preparation – towel up to expose the whole of the anterior neck
5. Skin – impress line of incision 3 cm above sternal notch with stout silk

Incision
Incise skin and platysma together in a collar incision 8 cm in length

Procedure
1. Elevate flaps of skin with platysma
   a. Superiorly to thyroid cartilage
   b. Inferiority to suprasternal notch
   c. Place Joll's retractor to retract skin flaps
2. Divide deep cervical fascia longitudinally in the midline
3. Separate strap muscles and retract laterally
4. Assess goitre
5. Ligate and divide in continuity (Fig. 6)
   a. Middle thyroid vein
   b. Superior thyroid vessels at the upper pole of the thyroid
6. Beware external laryngeal nerve
7. Identify and beware recurrent laryngeal nerve as it enters the operative field from below
8. Ligate and divide the branches of the inferior thyroid artery on the capsule of the gland (division laterally can embarrass the blood supply of the parathyroids)
9. Divide isthmus and place haemostats around margin of resection leaving 2 g of thyroid from each lobe
10. Identify and beware parathyroids

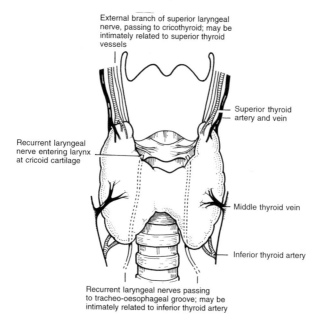

External branch of superior laryngeal
nerve, passing to cricothyroid; may be
intimately related to superior thyroid
vessels

Superior thyroid
artery and vein

Recurrent laryngeal
nerve entering larynx
at cricoid cartilage

Middle thyroid vein

Inferior thyroid artery

Recurrent laryngeal nerves passing
to tracheo-oesophageal groove; may be
intimately related to inferior thyroid artery

Fig. 6 Surgical anatomy of thyroid.

11. Any doubt as to whether yellow tissue is parathyroid or fat –
use the density test by placing in a jar of water. Parathyroid
tissue will sink slowly whereas fat will float on the surface
12. Repeat partial lobectomy on opposite side

Closure
1. Absolute haemostasis
2. Suction drain to thyroid bed
3. Close loosely in layers with absorbable sutures
4. Close the skin with sutures or clips
5. Check vocal cords on extubation by direct laryngoscopy

Postoperative management
Nursing
1. Half-hourly observation till conscious
2. At bed side
   a. Michel clip remover in case of respiratory distress due to
      haematoma
   b. 10 ml calcium gluconate 10% in case of acute hypocalcaemia
3. Keep semi-recumbent

Investigations
1. Review indirect laryngoscopy (especially if there is cord impairment on extubation)
2. Serum calcium regularly in the postoperative period
3. Thyroid function tests at 6 weeks postoperatively
4. Remove
   a. Drain when dry, 24–48 hours postoperatively
   b. Sutures/clips, 2–3 days postoperatively

Complications
1. Early
   a. Haemorrhage, usually reactionary
   b. Tetany
      • In first 3 days from corrected thyrotoxicosis
      • After 1 week with hypoparathyroidism
   c. Recurrent laryngeal nerve palsy
      • 95% neurapraxia and resolves
      • If bilateral, cords adduct to midline so needs immediate reintubation
   d. Thyroid crisis, if thyrotoxic patient is inadequately prepared, rare with modern techniques
2. Late
   a. Keloid scar
   b. Hypothyroidism – 20% of all patients undergoing partial thyroidectomy
   c. Recurrent thyrotoxicosis, <5% of patients undergoing thyroidectomy for Graves' disease

PRINCIPLES OF PARATHYROID SURGERY

Preoperative management of hyperparathyroidism
1. Reduce calcium intake, 500 mg daily calcium diet
2. Rehydrate orally or intravenously if severely hypercalcaemic (NB Steroids have no place in the management of hyperparathyroidism)
3. Exclude associated pathologies
   a. Those due to hypercalcaemia
      • Urinary tract stones
      • Duodenal ulcer
      • Pancreatitis
      • Psychosis
   b. Those associated with hyperparathyroidism
      • Chronic renal failure
   c. Those associated with parathyroid hyperplasia
      • Multiple endocrine neoplasia Type II
      • Medullary carcinoma thyroid
      • Phaeochromocytoma

d. Those associated with parathyroid adenoma
  - Multiple endocrine neoplasia Type I
  - Pancreatic endocrine tumours
  - Pituitary tumours

Parathyroid localisation studies

Method	Accuracy
Ultrasound (with aspiration cytology)	50–80% tumours of >0.5 cm
CT	>70% of tumours >1.0 cm
MRI	
Angiography – PTH venous sampling	Only lateralising
Selective arteriography	80%
Subtraction technetium thallium isotope scan	90%

Other tests
1. Group and save
2. Indirect laryngoscopy to assess vocal cords

Neck exploration
1. As for thyroidectomy (*see* p. 36)
2. Mobilise the thyroid by ligation and division of the middle thyroid veins
3. Fully explore both sides and account for all the parathyroids

Peroperative methods of parathyroid localisation
1. Methylene blue method, turns patient blue
2. Wang's density test, accurately differentiates adenomata from hyperplasia
3. Frozen section examination, needs an experienced parathyroid pathologist

Problems of parathyroid surgery
1. Localisation of all four glands
2. Common sites of ectopic glands
   a. Within the carotid sheath
   b. Retropharyngeal
   c. Within the thymus
   d. Within the thyroid (usually enveloped by a multinodular goitre)
   e. Superior mediastinum
3. Management of single versus multiple gland disease
   a. Single adenoma, excise
   b. Multiple adenoma, excise, leaving normal glands
   c. Hyperplasia, either excise $3^{1}/_{2}$ glands or total parathyroidectomy with forearm reimplantation of 100 mg of parathyroid tissue

Closure
As for thyroidectomy (see p. 36)

Postoperative management
1. Nurse semi recumbent and prepared to remove sutures at the first sign of respiratory embarrassment due to haematoma collection
2. Investigation
   a. Daily calcium estimation (if hypocalcaemic then correct with 1-α-calcidol (vitamin D) and oral or parenteral calcium)
   b. Histology of parathyroids
   c. Indirect laryngoscopy of vocal cords

Complications
1. Recurrent laryngeal nerve damage (as with thyroidectomy, see p. 36)
2. Hungry bone disease causing profound hypocalcaemia – rare, usually associated with parathyroid bone disease
3. Recurrent hypercalcaemia
   a. Inadequate excision or missed adenoma
   b. Other cause of hypercalcaemia (malignancy, sarcoid, etc.)

THYROGLOSSAL CYST AND FISTULA

Preoperative management
Special investigations, ultrasound of the neck

Pre-incision
1. General anaesthetic preferably with nasotracheal intubation
2. Position and skin preparation – as for thyroidectomy (see p. 36)

Incision
1. Cyst, transverse over cyst
2. Fistula, transverse elliptical around fistula opening

Procedure
1. Cyst
   a. Divide platysma in the line of the incision
   b. Divide the deep cervical fascia and strap muscle longitudinally in the midline over the cyst
   c. Excise the cyst
   d. Dissect out any fibrous track towards the hyoid bone as for a fistula (see below)
2. Fistula (Fig. 7)
   a. Sharply dissect out ascending fistula track as it passes between the strap muscles
   b. Elevate the upper skin flap with platysma to assist the dissection

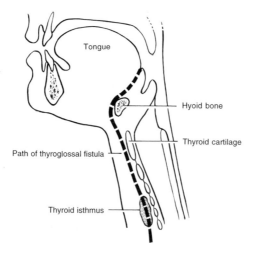

Fig. 7 Thyroglossal fistula.

c. Follow the fistula track up to the hyoid bone to which it is intimately related
d. Gently mobilise the body of the hyoid bone from its muscular attachment (mylohyoid, sternohyoid and thyrohyoid)
e. Excise the centre part of the body of hyoid en bloc with the fistula track
f. Follow and excise any remnant of the fistula track by dividing the median raphe of mylohyoid (it may continue as far as the foramen caecum of the tongue)
g. The final procedure can be aided by the assistant depressing the posterior tongue with his index finger

Closure
1. Absolute haemostasis
2. Suction drainage
3. Close in layers

Postoperative management
1. Remove the drain on the first postoperative day and sutures after 72 hours
2. Investigations, histological examination of the specimen

Complications
Recurrence of the fistula if inadequately excised or in the case of a thyroglossal abscess treated by simple drainage

EXCISION OF BRANCHIAL FISTULA

Preoperative management
1. Examine and exclude the presence of bilateral fistulae.
2. Warn the patient that the procedure may need several incisions
3. Investigations
   a. Lipoidal sinogram of track is optional
   b. Aspiration of branchial cyst shows cholesterol crystals on microscopy

Pre-incision
1. General anaesthesia with endotracheal intubation
2. Position – supine with the neck extended and the head turned slightly away
3. Skin preparation of lower face to upper chest
4. Towel up head separately and expose the whole of the lower face and neck on the affected side
5. Prior to incision, inject 3–5 ml of methylene blue into the fistula opening to delineate the track for dissection

Incision
1. Lower
   Elliptical in a skin crease around the fistula opening
2. Upper
   Transverse in a skin crease at the junction of the upper third and middle third of the neck over the anterior border of sternomastoid

Procedure
1. Sharply dissect out the lower fistula track en bloc with the fistula opening (this may be assisted with a probe lying in the track)
2. Dissect the track up towards the second incision deep to the platysma, elevating the skin flap off the fistula track
3. Pull the specimen through to the second incision and continue the dissection up to the point where it passes over the hypoglossal nerve
4. Continue the dissection of the track as it passes between
   a. External carotid artery anteriorly
   b. Internal carotid artery posteriorly to join the wall of the pharynx at the posterior fauces
5. Ligate the fistula track and excise the specimen

Closure
1. Absolute haemostasis
2. Suction drain
3. Close in layers

Postoperative management
1. Remove the drain when dry (24 hours)
2. Histology of fistula track

Complications
1. Uncommon
2. Incomplete excision may cause recurrence of a branchial cyst
3. Damage to hypoglossal nerve

EXCISION OF PHARYNGEAL POUCH

Preoperative management
1. Investigations
   a. Barium swallow
   b. Oesophagoscopy (there is a risk of perforation of the pouch with careless instrumentation)
2. Chest physiotherapy, since often these patients are elderly with a history of aspiration of pouch contents

Pre-incision
1. General anaesthesia and endotracheal intubation
2. Position – supine
3. Prior to towelling up, perform direct pharyngoscopy and pack the pouch either by the traditional method of a half-inch ribbon gauze dyed with flavine or with the inflated balloon of a Foley catheter
4. Skin preparation of mouth to nipples and towel up to expose all of the neck

Incision
1. On the side to which the pouch is directed (90% to the left)
2. Transverse across the lower third of sternomastoid on the affected side

Procedure
1. Divide the deep cervical fascia along the anterior border of sternomastoid and retract the muscle posteriorly
2. Divide the tendinous mid-point of omohyoid to expose the carotid sheath
3. Ligate and divide middle thyroid vein and the inferior thyroid artery if it crosses the operative field
4. Gently retract
   a. Thyroid medially
   b. Carotid sheath laterally thus exposing the pouch
5. Mobilise the pouch in the neck by sharp dissection and when it is free, remove the pre-placed pack or balloon

6. Excise the sac at its neck, flush with the pharyngeal wall between thyropharyngeus superiorly and cricopharyngeus inferiorly
7. Perform a cricopharyngeus myotomy
8. Close the pharyngeal defect in two layers

Closure
1. Place
   a. Fine bore soft nasogastric feeding tube
   b. Suction type drain to the wound
2. Close in layers

Postoperative management
1. Remove the drains when dry at 24–48 hours
2. Feed via nasogastric tube from first postoperative day
3. Barium swallow at the 5th postoperative day to check the pharyngeal closure; allow to eat and drink if there is no leakage

Complications
1. Pharyngeal fistula
2. Recurrent pouch (if the excision is inadequate)

BLOCK DISSECTION TO THE NECK

Indications
1. Lymph node metastases from primary head malignancies, especially
   a. Carcinoma of the lip, floor of mouth, tongue and skin
   b. Malignant melanoma
2. Thyroid malignancy
   a. Papillary
   b. Medullary
3. Salivary malignancy
4. Lymph node recurrence after radiotherapy to cervical node metastases
5. Tuberculosis with the failure of chemotherapy and the absence of suppuration

Anatomical consideration of dissection (Fig. 8)
1. To remove the structure of the digastric triangle
   a. Submandibular gland
   b. Submandibular nodes
2. To remove internal jugular vein (IJV)
3. To remove deep cervical chain of lymph node
   a. Upper anterior sternomastoid group
   b. Upper posterior sternomastoid group
   c. Lower anterior sternomastoid group
   d. Lower posterior sternomastoid group
4. To remove sternocleidomastoid node

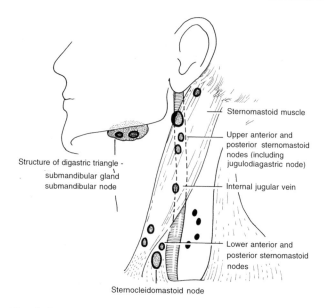

Structure of digastric triangle -
    submandibular gland
    submandibular node

Sternomastoid muscle

Upper anterior and
posterior sternomastoid
nodes (including
jugulodiagastric node)

Internal jugular vein

Lower anterior and
posterior sternomastoid
nodes

Sternocleidomastoid node

Fig. 8 Structures to remove at radical block dissection of neck.

Preoperative management – determine primary pathology
1. Clinical examination
2. Endoscopy with biopsy/brush cytology
3. Radiology
    a. Primary pathology
    b. Bone involvement
    c. Contrast studies
    d. Lymphangiogram
    e. CT
4. Skin test
    a. Heaf/Mantoux for TB
    b. Kveim for sarcoid
5. Sputum
    a. Cytology
    b. Culture/AFBs
6. Fine needle aspiration cytology

Pre-incision
1. General anaesthesia with endotracheal intubation
2. Position – supine with neck extended and head turned away
3. Skin preparation of mid face to lower chest, towelled up to expose all of neck
4. Mark out skin incision with a marker pen

Incision
Semicircular. Commence at the midline just below the mandible and descend curving outwards to a point on the lateral border sternomastoid 2 cm above the clavicle and then curve upwards to the mastoid process, including platysma with the skin

Procedure
1. Ligate and divide the external jugular vein
2. Elevate the skin flap with platysma for the whole width of the incision to the top of the neck
3. Divide the origin of sternomastoid 2.5 cm above the clavicle and retract upwards to expose the internal jugular vein in the carotid sheath
4. Ligate and divide the internal jugular vein at the root of the neck
5. Gently dissect the internal jugular vein, deep cervical lymph nodes and sternomastoid en bloc off the carotid artery
6. Beware
   a. Vagus nerve between the IJV and the carotid artery
   b. Phrenic nerve appearing from behind the scalenus anterior in the posterior triangle
   c. Thoracic duct on left
   d. Hypoglossal nerve crossing the external and internal carotid arteries laterally above the carotid bifurcation, and giving off the descendens hypoglossi
7. Ligate and divide any branches of the IJV in the neck, especially the common facial vein
8. Continue the dissection to the base of the skull and ligate and divide the origin of the IJV, excise the mastoid head of sternomastoid and remove the specimen enbloc
9. The dissection may continue into the anterior triangle to include the contents of the digastric triangle

Closure
1. Meticulous haemostasis
2. 1 or 2 suction drains
3. Apposition of platysma
4. Close the skin with interrupted sutures

Postoperative management
1. Continue suction drainage for several days until the drainage is minimal
2. Histological examination of the specimen

Complications

1. Early
   a. Seroma under the skin flap
   b. Skin flap necrosis, especially with incisions which involve the apposition of three or more skin flaps
   c. Raised intracranial pressure uncommon, only occurs with simultaneous bilateral block dissections
2. Late
   Disease recurrence

Cardiothoracic surgery

OESOPHAGOSCOPY AND DILATATION

Preoperative management
1. Investigations
   a. Barium swallow
   b. Chest X-ray
   c. Group and save for dilatation
2. Warn patient of the possible risk of oesophageal perforation

Pre-procedure
1. Local anaesthetic lignocaine spray to throat
2. i.v. sedation using benzodiazepine plus i.v. opioid analgesia (e.g. pethidine)
3. Position – lateral
4. Surgeon stands beside the patient's head, wearing protective glasses
5. Protect the patient's eyes with a towel
6. Pulse oximeter

Procedure
1. Pass the oesophagoscope to the back of the oropharynx. Visualize the epiglottis and cords
2. Gently pass the 'scope through cricopharyngeus
3. Now pass the 'scope gently to the stricture
4. Be very careful
   a. With patients with rheumatoid arthritis when extending the neck (all should have a preoperative cervical spine X-ray. *See* Principles of surgery for rheumatoid arthritis, p. 181)
   b. With patients with osteoarthritis who may have severe thoracic spine osteophytes (who should have a preoperative lateral chest X-ray)
5. Visualise the pathology
   a. Biopsy/brush cytology
   b. Dilate the stricture
   c. Dilators
      • Eder–Peustow
      • Celestin

6. Dilatation
   a. Pass the guide wire through the stricture under direct vision
   b. Remove the 'scope carefully over the guide wire
   c. Pass the dilator gently over the guide wire and through the stricture
   d. Repeat, if necessary using wider dilators
7. Remove the 'scope

Postoperative management
Chest X-ray following dilatation, to exclude oesophageal perforation, the patient must remain nil by mouth until this is seen and reported as normal by the surgeon

Complications
1. Oesophageal perforation
2. Aspiration (especially after intubation of a low oesophageal stricture)
3. Recurrent stricture

RIGID BRONCHOSCOPY

Preoperative management
1. Chest X-rays
   a. PA and lateral
   b. Tomography of lesion
   c. (CT)
2. Sputum
   a. Culture
   b. AFBs
   c. Cytology
3. Skin testing
   a. Heaf test
   b. Kveim test
Preoperative physiotherapy with mucolytics and bronchodilators in chronic obstructive airways disease (*see* Principles of prevention and treatment of pulmonary problems during operations, p. 9)

Pre-procedure
1. General anaesthetic
2. Position – supine with shoulders supported, neck in neutral position and the head flexed on the neck
3. Surgeon standing behind the patient's head wearing protective glasses
4. Towel placed to protect the patient's eyes

Procedure
1. Select a bronchoscope of appropriate size (large adult, small adult, child, infant, neonate)

2. Once anaesthetic has been induced pass the 'scope over the back of the tongue and extend the head on the neck. Depress the larynx with the left hand, passing the scope behind the epiglottis under direct vision to see the vocal cords
3. Gently pass the 'scope through the vocal cords into the trachea
4. Negotiate down the trachea to the carina and measure its distance from the teeth
5. Visualise the normal bronchial tree first by passing the 'scope down the main bronchus and using angled telescopes to look into the major segment bronchi
6. Now visualise the abnormal bronchial tree, repeating the procedure
   a. Take brush cytology/biopsy specimens
   b. Remove foreign material/bodies
   c. Trap sputum
   • Cytology
   • Culture
7. Remove the 'scope

Preoperative management
Obtain results from specimens removed

Complications
Haemoptysis
1. Rough handling
2. Biopsy of vascular lesion

POSTEROLATERAL THORACOTOMY
Preoperative management
1. Commence physiotherapy and breathing exercises
2. Examine and mark the side, shave the chest and axilla
3. Investigations relevant to the pathology
   a. Chest X-ray (PA and lateral)
   b. Cross-match blood appropriate to procedure
   c. Bronchoscopy results
   d. Oesophagoscopy
   e. Mediastinoscopy
4. Prophylactic antibiotics, ampicillin and flucloxacillin
5. Intravenous infusion
6. Catheter

Pre-incision
1. General anaesthetic with a double lumen endotracheal tube (e.g. Robertshaw)
2. Position
   Lateral, with upper arm supported and the patient's back perpendicular to the edge of the operating table, support the upper leg with a pillow

3. Skin preparation of all of back from the nape of the neck to the small of the back and extending to the midline at the front
4. Towel up to expose the posterior and subaxillary hemithorax

Incision (Fig. 9)
Commence 8 cm lateral to the 6th thoracic spinous process and curve forward, 2 cm below the tip of the scapula to the mid axillary line in the line of the ribs

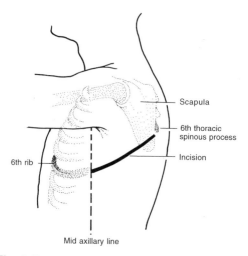

Fig. 9 Posterolateral thoracotomy incision.

Procedure
1. With the cutting diathermy divide
   a. Latissimus dorsi
   b. Serratus anterior in the line of the incision
2. Retract the lower scapula and count the ribs by palpation from the top (the uppermost being the 2nd rib) as far as the 6th rib
3. Elevate the periosteum of the 6th rib for the length of the incision and clear the periosteum completely off the circumference of the posterior 3 cm of the rib with Doyen's periosteal elevator
4. Divide the posterior end of the rib with a bone cutter and elevate the rib from its periosteal bed via its superior edge (reducing the risk of damage to the intercostal neurovascular bundle)
5. Gently insert the rib spreader and open slowly, picking up the parietal pleura to open it, allowing the lung to fall away
6. Open the rib spreader and divide any pleural adhesions
7. Assess the pleural cavity and carry out the procedure

Closure
1. Haemostasis, swab and instrument check
2. Place two pleural drains
   a. Apical for air
   b. Basal for blood and connect to underwater seal drainage systems
3. Insert an intercostal nerve block with 0.5% Marcain for the intercostal space of entry and the two spaces above and below
4. Close in layers

Postoperative management
1. Chest X-ray in recovery, and then daily until the chest drains are removed to assess lung expansion
2. Nurse in a sitting position and commence postoperative physiotherapy on the same day
3. Place the pleural drains on a low pressure suction pump for at least 24 hours and until the lung is fully up (5 cm water pressure on a Roberts pump)
4. Remove the drain when the lung is up, no air is being drained and the fluid drainage is less than 100 ml daily
5. Methods of analgesia
   a. Marcain intercostal block
   b. High thoracic opiate epidural
   c. Intravenous opiate infusion

Complications
1. Early
   a. Infection
      • Wound
      • Septicaemia
      • Respiratory
      • Emphysema
   b. Pneumothorax
   c. Surgical emphysema
   d. Haemothorax
2. Late
   a. Chronic suppuration
   b. Intercostal neuroma

MEDIAN STERNOTOMY

Indications
1. Cardiac surgery
2. Surgery of the superior mediastinum (thymectomy, retrosternal thyroidectomy, surgery of the trachea and paratracheal nodes)

Preoperative management
1. Investigations
   a. Chest X-ray (PA and lateral)
   b. Cardiac investigations relevant to pathology (*see* Principles of cardiac surgery, p. 58)
   c. Bronchoscopy prior to tracheal surgery (*see* Rigid bronchoscopy, p. 50)
2. Examine the legs and mark the long saphenous vein prior to coronary artery bypass graft surgery (*see* Principles of cardiac surgery, p. 58)
3. Prophylactic antibiotics, ampicillin and flucloxacillin
4. Intravenous line
5. Central venous catheter
6. Arterial pressure monitor
7. Bladder catheter

Pre-incision
1. General anaesthesia and endotracheal intubation
2. Position — supine
3. Skin preparation of upper neck to lower abdomen, towel up to expose sternum

Incision
Midline from the suprasternal notch to just below the xiphoid process

Procedure
1. Divide the subcutaneous tissues to the sternal periosteum with diathermy point, including the linea alba immediately below the xiphisternum
2. Bluntly dissect the tissues immediately behind the xiphoid
3. Divide the sternum longitudinally with a mechanical reciprocating saw
4. Beware the pleura overlapping the mediastinum anteriorly which may be inadvertently opened
5. Insert a self-retaining retractor and gently open to display the pericardium inferiorly and the great vessels superiorly
6. Perform appropriate surgery

Closure
1. Meticulous haemostasis
2. Place two pericardial drains and bring them out below the xiphoid through separate incisions in the rectus sheath
3. Pass steel wire sutures (5 metric gauge) around the sternum and twist closed to give an accurate closure
4. Close the linea alba
5. Close the subcutaneous tissues and skin in layers

Postoperative management
1. Chest X-ray in the recovery ward – exclude pneumothorax
2. Nurse on intensive care unit after cardiac surgery and continue ventilation at the discretion of the anaesthetist
3. Remove the pericardial drains when the drainage is minimal (< 50 ml in 24 hours)
4. Check the haemoglobin and transfuse accordingly

Complications
1. Early
   a. Pneumothorax
   b. Haemothorax
   c. Pericardial tamponade
   d. Those specific to cardiac surgery (*see* Principles of cardiac surgery, p. 58)
   e. Sternal dehiscence
2. Late
   Keloid scar

PNEUMONECTOMY

Indications
Malignant lung tumours not amenable to lobectomy

Preoperative management
As for posterolateral thoracotomy (*see* p. 51)
1. Examine the patient, mark the side and pulmonary function tests
2. Chest X-ray (PA and lateral)
3. Tomography
4. (CT)
5. Sputum
   a. Microbiology
   b. Cytology
6. Bronchoscopy (fibreoptic/rigid *see* p. 50)
   a. Cytology
   b. Histology
7. Metastases
   Liver
   a. Function tests
   b. Ultrasound
   Bone
   a. Skeletal survey
   b. Isotope bone scan
   Nodes
   a. Chest CT
   b. Mediastinoscopy

Indications of inoperability
1. Evidence of metastases (including tracheal nodes)
2. Tumours <2 cm from carina
3. Patient >70 years old requiring a pneumonectomy
4. Nerve involvement
   a. Recurrent laryngeal
   b. Phrenic
   c. Pancoast syndrome – T1 – Horner's syndrome
5. Chest wall/diaphragm invaded
6. SVC obstruction

Relative contraindications
1. Blood stained pleural effusion
2. Poor respiratory reserve on pulmonary function tests (FVC, FEV, peak flow and blood gases)

Pre-incision
(See Posterolateral thoracotomy, p. 51)

Procedure
1. Allow the lung to collapse away from the parietal pleura and assess the tumour (pleural, hilar and lymph node spread). It may be necessary to open the pericardium to fully assess the operability of the tumour
2. Divide the pulmonary ligament to mobilise the lung, open the hilar pleura anteriorly
3. Gently dissect out, ligate and divide the pulmonary veins
4. Very carefully dissect, ligate and divide the branches of the pulmonary artery lying anterior to the main bronchus
5. Finally clamp and divide the bronchus, closing this with interrupted monofilament nylon or steel sutures
6. Remove the specimen for histological examination
7. Dissect out the subcarinal and peritracheal lymph nodes for histological examination

Closure
1. Close the pleura over the hilar stump
2. Crush the phrenic nerve, allowing the diaphragm to elevate to occupy the pleural space
3. No drains
4. Close in layers (see Posterolateral thoracotomy, p. 51)

Postoperative management
(See Posterolateral thoracotomy, p. 51)
1. Check the intra pleural pressure in the recovery room using an anaeroid manometer and two-way tap, adjust to atmospheric pressure
2. Nurse in a sitting position

Investigations
1. Chest X-ray
2. Histology of tumour and lymph nodes

Complications
1. Early
   a. Secretion retention
   b. Surgical emphysema
   c. Pericardial cardiac herniation
   d. Empyema
   e. Bronchopleural fistula
2. Late
   Tumour recurrence (75% of cases)

DRAINAGE OF EMPYEMA

Pathological factors
An empyema is a pleural abscess, not just the presence of pus within the pleural cavity (pyothorax). Formal drainage should not be undertaken until an empyema is established, pyothorax should be treated by aspiration, local antibiotic instillation and systemic antibiotics

Preoperative management
1. Establish diagnosis
   a. Clinical examination
   b. Chest X-ray (PA and lateral)
   c. Needle aspiration (pus for microbiological examination)
2. Exclude bronchopleural fistula (suggested by an air fluid level on the chest X-ray)
3. Antibiotic cover determined by microbiological results

Pre-incision
1. Anaesthesia with local anaesthetic with mild sedation
2. Position – sitting, with access to the back (most empyemas lie posteriorly)
3. Skin preparation of the whole of the posterior hemithorax and towel up to expose a large area overlying the empyema

Incision
Decide from the chest X-rays which rib overlies the empyema and incise directly over it for 8 cm

Procedure
1. Deepen in the line of the skin incision
2. Infiltrate the periosteum of the rib and intercostal nerve with local anaesthetic
3. Divide the periosteum and elevate this to expose the rib

4. Excise 3 cm of rib and ligate the intercostal vessels at each end of the excision
5. Excise a wide disc of thickened pleura and suck out any free pus, sending a further specimen for microbiological examination
6. Gently, digitally break down any loculi and remove any solid debris with ovum forceps
7. Insert a wide bore silastic chest drain and close the wound around it, securing the drain to the skin
8. Connect the drain to an underwater seal drainage system with low pressure suction (<5 cm water)

Postoperative management
1. Chest X-ray in recovery ward
2. After a few days cut off the drain 2–3 cm from the skin and leave on open, free drainage
3. Daily physiotherapy
4. Review collapse of the cavity with regular sinograms

Complications
1. Bronchopleural fistula from traumatic tube insertion
2. Fibrous cortex to cavity – therefore, does not collapse and needs decortication

PRINCIPLES OF CARDIAC SURGERY
Preoperation
1. Diagnosis with
   a. Echocardiography
   b. Angiography
   c. Electrocardiography
2. Treat co-existing disease
   a. Pulmonary
   b. Diabetes
   c. Peripheral vascular disease, especially carotid pathology
3. Check electrolytes, especially potassium (diuretics, infusion, dilution)
4. Anaesthetic
   a. Avoid excessive O_2 demand
   b. Decrease sympathetic activity
   c. Increase PaO_2

Peroperative
1. Hypothermia
   a. Systemic
   b. Pericardial
2. Approach heart via median sternotomy (*see* p. 53)

3. Cardiopulmonary bypass (extra corporeal circulation)
   a. Needs heparinisation, which is reversed at the end by protamine
   b. Gas and heat interchange
   c. Arrest heart in diastole (myocardium is at maximal relaxation)
   d. Cardioplegia
      • Cold
      • Potassium chloride (e.g. St Thomas' solution)
   e. Drain venae cavae to the pump and return blood to the aortic arch
   f. Cross clamp the aortic root (decreases the loss of cardioplegic drugs and blood)
   g. Cardiovent at the end of the procedure
   h. Remove air
   i. Reduce blood transfusion requirement by using aprotinin and haemodilution
4. During the procedure, monitor
   a. Serum potassium
   b. PaO_2 (> 10 KPa)
   c. Urine output (> 1 ml/minute)
   d. Mean arterial pressure (> 60 mmHg)

Post surgery
Monitor
   1. Pulse and arterial pressure
   2. ECG
   3. Central venous pressure
   4. Urine output
   5. Potassium
   6. Blood gases on ventilation

VALVE SURGERY

Indications for surgery
   1. Failure of medical treatment
   2. Regurgitation with poor compensation

Methods
1. Valvotomy
   a. Closed
   b. Open
2. Plastic repair of valve
3. Mechanical valve replacement, e.g. Starr Edwards (ball and cage), Bjork Shilley (tilting disc)

a. Advantages
   - Convenience
   - Easily sewn in
   - Durability
   Therefore useful for younger patients
   b. Disadvantages
   - Clotting
   - Embolisation
4. Biological valve replacement
   a. Cadaveric homograft
      Advantage
      - No clotting problems
      Disadvantages
      - Limited supply
      - Difficult implantation
      - 'Wears out', usually within 8 years
   b. Porcine xenograft
      Advantages
      - Good supply
      - Glutaraldehyde treatment sterilises the graft and
        strengthens the structure
      - Easier to suture in place
      - Minimal risk of embolism (therefore does not need
        warfarin)
      Disadvantage
      - Calcify, especially in younger children

Operative mortality
1. Single valve – 5–8% (8–10% if combined with coronary artery
   bypass graft)
2. Multiple valve – 10–12%

Complications of valve replacement
1. Thrombosis
2. Embolism
   a. Vegetation
   b. Valve
      - In part
      - All of valve
3. Infection
   a. Early – *Staphylococcus*
   b. Late – *Streptococcus viridans*
4. Paravalvular leak

SURGERY FOR CORONARY ARTERY DISEASE

Indications
1. Disabling angina despite full medical treatment, including balloon angioplasty with proximal arterial (> 70%) stenosis
2. Crescendo angina
3. Post myocardial infarction
   a. Left ventricular aneurysm
   b. Ventriculo septal defect
   c. Ruptured papillary muscle

Preoperative investigations
1. Exclude life threatening peripheral vascular disease, especially carotid pathology
2. Blood
   a. Lipids/cholesterol
   b. Blood sugar
   c. Plasma viscosity/packed cell volume
3. ECG and stress ECG studies
4. Angiography
   a. Proximal stenosis
   b. Stenosis >70%
5. Echocardiography
6. Mark out saphenous vein

Method
1. Dissect out saphenous vein, ligating all branches and marking the direction of blood flow
2. Median sternotomy to expose the heart and initiate cardiopulmonary bypass with cardioplegia
3. Perform vein bypasses from aorta (side-to-end anastomosis) to distal coronary artery (end-to-side anastomosis). Reversing the vein
4. Other methods
   a. Endarterectomy (proximal short stenosis)
   b. Single snake graft with multiple anastomoses
   c. Internal mammary coronary anastomosis

Operative mortality – 4%
Results
1. Asymptomatic – 70%
2. Improvement in angina – 12%
3. No improvement – 13%
4. Early death – 4%
5. Late death – 3%

Complications
1. Peroperative infarction
2. Stroke
   a. Unsuspected carotid stenosis
   b. Embolism
3. Late graft occlusion

REPAIR OF AORTIC COARCTATION

Indications for surgery
1. Infancy
   a. Left ventricular failure
   b. In combination with surgery for other anomalies
2. Children
   Before 6 years old and onset of hypertension

Preoperative management
1. Correct congestive cardiac failure and hypertension as much as is possible (although in an emergency this must not postpone surgery)
2. Investigations
   a. Aortography
      • Delineate coarctation
      • Pressure gradient studies
      • Exclude patent ductus arteriosus
   b. Echocardiography
      • Exclude co-existent aortic and mitral valve abnormalities
   c. ECG
      • Left ventricular hypertrophy
   d. CXR
      • May show rib notching in older children
3. Broad spectrum antibiotic prophylaxis
4. Continuous monitor
   a. IVI
   b. CVP
   c. Pulmonary wedge pressure
   d. Arterial pressure
   e. ECG
   f. Catheterise bladder

Pre-incision
1. General anaesthesia with double lumen endotracheal tube to allow collapse of left lung. Careful peroperative control of blood pressure with sodium nitro-prusside
2. Perform an extended left posterolateral thoracotomy (*see* p. 51)
3. Beware distended chest wall collateral vessels

Procedure
1. Divide the mediastinal pleura vertically from the left subclavian artery to well below the coarctation
2. Identify the vagus nerve overlying aortic arch
3. Ligate and divide the left superior intercostal vein
4. Mobilise the left subclavian artery, distal aortic arch, coarctation and descending aorta and place slings around these vessels
5. Ligate and divide the ligamentum/ductus arteriosum
6. Beware the left recurrent laryngeal nerve arching under aorta
7. Place clamps to control the aorta above and below the coarctation
8. Excise the coarctation and perform an end-to-end anastomosis to repair the aorta
9. Problems
   a. Long coarctation
      • Dacron patch aortoplasty
      • Dacron tube graft
   b. Infantile preductal coarctation
      • Subclavian flap operation
   c. Inadequate collateral circulation impairs peroperative renal perfusion (pressure in descending aorta <<50 mm Hg) – use left atriofemoral bypass

Closure
1. Repair the parietal pleura
2. Close as posterolateral thoracotomy (*see* p. 51)

Postoperative management
1. Monitor in an intensive care unit until stable
2. Monitor cardiac function
   a. Arterial pressure
   b. CVP
   c. Pulmonary wedge pressure
   d. ECG
3. Monitor renal function
   a. Output
   b. Electrolytes
   c. Osmolality

Operative mortality
1. Infant with other anomalies >10%
2. Childhood – 2%
3. Adult – 2–5%

Complications
1. Early
   a. Haemorrhage (especially chest wall collaterals)
   b. Recurrent laryngeal nerve palsy

c. Chylothorax
d. Paraplegia
e. Acute renal failure
2. Late
  a. Persistent hypertension (if longstanding coarctation resulted in renal changes)
  b. Recurrent coarctation

CLOSURE OF PATENT DUCTUS ARTERIOSUS

Indications for surgery
1. Left ventricular failure
2. Aneurysmal dilatation of the ductus
3. Bacterial endocarditis

Contraindications for surgery
Severe pulmonary hypertension with shunt reversal

Preoperative management
1. Cardiac catheterisation
  a. Confirm diagnosis
  b. Exclude coexistent abnormalities
  c. Measure pulmonary vascular resistance
2. Timing of surgery
  a. Ideally between age 2–5 years
  b. Onset of complications
3. Broad spectrum antibiotic prophylaxis
4. IVI
5. Catheterise
6. Systemic and pulmonary arterial pressure monitor
7. ECG monitor

Pre-incision
1. General anaesthesia with double lumen endotracheal intubation to allow deflation of the left lung
2. Perform left lateral thoracotomy (see p. 51)

Procedure
1. Allow the lung to collapse and retract it forwards
2. Incise the mediastinal pleura overlying the aorta from proximal to the origin of the left subclavian artery to below the ductus which can be palpated as a thrill
3. Gently mobilise the aorta and place tapes proximally and distally
4. Retraction on the tapes displays the ductus, left vagus and left recurrent laryngeal nerve passing under the ductus

5. Test clamp the ductus
   If there is no fall in pulmonary artery pressure then abandon the operation
6. Doubly ligate the ductus with a non-absorbable suture

Closure
Close the parietal pleura (*see* Posterolateral thoracotomy, p. 51)

Postoperative management
1. Nurse on an intensive care unit until stable
2. Investigate pulmonary artery pressures

Complications
Operative mortality
1. Children without pulmonary hypertension – 0.5%
2. Children with pulmonary hypertension and adults – 1.0%
Ductus recanalisation <0.1%

PRINCIPLES OF OESOPHAGECTOMY

Indications
1. Adenocarcinoma of the cardia or arising within ectopic gastric mucosa (Barrett's oesophagus)
2. Squamous carcinoma of the oesophagus (results are comparable with radiotherapy)
3. Benign oesophageal stricture not amenable to dilatation and anti-reflux procedures

Pathological factors
1. 70% of malignancies are squamous carcinomas
2. 30% of malignancies are adenocarcinomas (either arising in a Barrett's oesophagus or at the cardia)
3. Direct spread is early since the oesophagus has no serosa and submucosal spread is extensive
4. Lymphatic spread is early
5. Sites of tumours
   a. Upper third – 15%
   b. Middle third – 50%
   c. Lower third – 35%
6. Because of dysphagia these patients are often in a poor state of nutrition at presentation

Preoperative management
1. Investigations
   a. Barium swallow
   b. Chest X-ray
   c. Oesophagoscopy and biopsy (*see* p. 49)

   d. Bronchoscopy for tumours of upper and mid third (*see* p. 50)
to exclude tracheal involvement
   e. Chest CT – involvement of adjacent structures and lymph
nodes
   f. Endoscopic ultrasonography
   g. Liver metastases
     • Liver function tests
     • Ultrasound
2. If malnourished, then correct the catabolic effect for at least 10
days prior to surgery
   a. Enterally
     • Nasogastric tube
     • Gastrostomy
   b. Parenterally
3. Chest physiotherapy
4. Bowel preparation (*see* p. 104) if colonic interposition anticipated
5. Antibiotic prophylaxis; broad spectrum (metronidazole if colonic
interposition anticipated)
6. IVI
7. Catheter
8. CVP monitor

TUMOUR AT 35–40 CM FROM THE TEETH

1. Use a left thoracoabdominal incision
2. The limit to this approach is the arch of the aorta which crosses
the mid third of the oesophagus
3. Position – left semilateral

Incision
Oblique, commencing to the right of the midline in the epigastrium
and up to the left costal margin and extended via the bed of the left
7th rib posteriorly to the posterior axillary line

Procedure
1. Full laparotomy, exclude liver and peritoneal metastases
2. Divide the diaphragm circumferentially to protect the
innervation of the phrenic nerve
3. Mobilise the stomach by dividing the left gastric vessels, short
gastric vessels and left gastroepiploic vessels
4. Divide the left pulmonary ligament to improve access to the
oesophagus
5. Mobilise the lower third of the oesophagus
6. Resect the specimen
7. Reconstruction for squamous carcinoma of the lower third
   a. Resect only the upper half of the stomach and anastomose
the distal gastric remnant to the lower oesophagus
   b. If the gap is too great then manage as (8)

8. Reconstruction for adenocarcinoma
   a. Perform partial proximal gastrectomy
   b. Anastomose distal stomach to the oesophagus

Closure
1. Drain the anastomoses and the left pleural space
2. Close in layers

TUMOUR AT 25–35 CM FROM THE TEETH

1. Use the Ivor Lewis method
2. Position – initially supine
3. Perform an upper midline incision and a full laparotomy (exclude liver and peritoneal metastases)
4. Mobilise the upper stomach (divide left gastric, short gastric and left gastroepiploic vessels)
5. Close the abdominal incision
6. Place in right lateral position
7. Perform a right posterolateral thoracotomy (*see* p. 51)
8. Divide the right pulmonary ligament and the azygos vein as it crosses the oesophagus
9. Gently mobilise the oesophagus and tumour and pull through the proximal stomach into the chest
10. Resect the tumour
11. Anastomose the proximal stomach to the upper oesophagus

Closure
1. Drain the anastomosis and the right pleural space
2. Close in layers (*see* Posterolateral thoracotomy, p. 51)

TUMOUR AT 15–25 CM FROM THE TEETH

May be managed palliatively by radiotherapy alone
50 Gy in fractions over 4–5 weeks

Operation
1. Use the McKeown method
2. First two stages as for the Ivor Lewis method without resection within the chest

Third stage
The third stage of the procedure is a right cervical incision and mobilisation of the cervical oesophagus from which the oesophageal specimen is withdrawn, delivering the proximal stomach to the neck

Resection
Resect the tumour and anastomose the proximal stomach to the hypopharynx

Closure
1. Drain
   a. Cervical anastomosis
   b. Right pleural space
2. Close in layers

Alternative method
1. Replace the oesophagus with mobilised transverse colon based on a pedicle of left upper colic artery supported by the marginal artery, lying either in the oesophageal bed, retrosternally or subcutaneously presternally, this needs
   a. Preoperative bowel preparation (see p. 104)
   b. Antibiotic prophylaxis for Gram-negative organisms and anaerobes
   c. A further anastomosis, mobilising the right hemicolon and anastomosing it to the left hemicolon

POSTOPERATIVE MANAGEMENT

Investigations
1. Chest X-ray in recovery: exclude a pneumothorax in the opposite hemithorax to that which has been operated on
2. Histology of specimen
3. Barium swallow at 5 days post surgery
   Anastomosis
   a. Patency
   b. Leaks
   c. Gastric emptying, since truncal vagotomy is inevitable with oesophagectomy

Remove drains when swallowing normally with no leaks from anastomosis

Consider parenteral nutrition in postoperative phase

Complications
1. Early
   a. Respiratory problems common (see p. 10)
   b. Anastomotic leakage and fistulae
   c. Pneumothorax
2. Late
   a. Anastomotic stricture
      • Fibrous
      • Tumour recurrence
   b. Distant tumour recurrence

3. Mortality
   a. Operative 10–20%
   b. 5-year survival <15%
4. Inoperable tumour
   a. Locally fixed squamous carcinoma then treat with
      radiotherapy
   b. Metastatic squamous carcinoma or adenocarcinoma –
      consider palliative intubation to relieve dysphagia
      Endoscopically placed tube
      • Atkinson's modification of Celestin's tube
      • Souttar's tube
        Surgically placed tube
      • Celestin's tube
      • Mousseau–Barbin's tube
      (Many other tubes are commercially available)

Upper gastrointestinal surgery

HELLER'S OPERATION FOR ACHALASIA

Indications for surgery
1. Failure of conservative treatment (hydrostatic dilatation)
2. Worsening dysphagia
3. Secondary organic changes within the oesophagus (ulceration)
4. Pulmonary complications (repeated aspiration)

Preoperative management
1. Investigations
   a. Barium swallow
   b. Oesophagoscopy and biopsy to exclude malignant stricture
   c. Oesophageal manometry
2. Correct nutritional status, since these patients are often malnourished at the time of presentation
3. Aspirate the oesophagus and chest physiotherapy as there is a significant risk of aspiration of oesophageal contents
4. IVI
5. Nasogastric tube

Pre-incision
1. General anaesthesia with endotracheal intubation
2. Position – supine
3. Skin preparation for an upper abdominal incision

Incision
Upper midline or laparoscopic approach

Procedure
1. Full laparotomy/laparoscopy, examine the cardia to exclude any other causes of dysphagia
2. Retract the left lobe of the liver medially (with or without division of the left triangular ligament) to expose the abdominal oesophagus

3. Divide the peritoneum overlying the oesophagus and gently mobilise the oesophagus. Place a sling around the oesophagus
4. Divide the transverse vessels at the cardia between ligatures
5. Commence the myotomy immediately below the cardia on the anterior stomach and extend it upwards longitudinally on the anterior oesophagus to the point where it is clearly dilated (Fig. 10)
6. Beware anterior vagus nerve – lying on oesophagus
   a. Damage during oesophageal traction to
      • Left gastric vessels
      • Short gastric vessel
      • Spleen
   b. Perforating the mucosa during seromyotomy (close with absorbable suture and non-suction drain)
7. Suture the fundus of the stomach to the left and then the right edges of the myotomy folding the fundus across anteriorly (Dor® procedure)
8. Closure
   a. Haemostasis
   b. No drains if no mucosal breach
   c. Close abdomen in layers

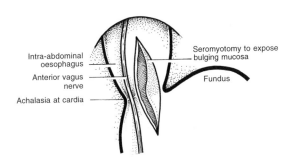

Fig. 10 Heller's seromyotomy for achalasia.

Postoperative management
1. Remove the nasogastric tube and commence oral fluids the next day (wait 48–72 hours if mucosal breach)
2. Investigations only if symptoms persist, then repeat investigations for achalasia
3. Complications (early)
   a. Peritonitis with missed mucosal perforation
   b. Persistent dysphagia – either oedema from manipulation at surgery or incomplete myotomy
   c. Reactionary haemorrhage from spleen or short gastric vessels

SURGERY FOR GASTRO-OESOPHAGEAL REFLUX AND HIATUS HERNIA

Aim of surgery
To restore and maintain an intra-abdominal segment of oesophagus

Indications for surgery
1. Gastro-oesophageal reflux
   a. Failure of medical treatment for intractible symptoms
   b. Complications
      • Peptic ulcer
      • Peptic stricture
      • Carcinoma
      • Haemorrhage
      • Recurrent aspiration
2. Sliding hiatus hernia if associated with indications to operate for gastro-oesophageal reflux
3. Rolling hiatus hernia almost always should be operated because of the risk of strangulation of either the fundus or small bowel within the sac and the associated risk of gastric volvulus

Principles of surgery
1. Restore intra-abdominal oesophagus
2. Create an oesophageal 'valve' or 'flap'
3. Perform repair of hiatus around a soft oesophageal bougie or tube, so it is not too tight
4. Preserve vagi
5. Investigations
   a. Chest X-ray
   b. Barium swallow
   c. Oesophagoscopy and biopsy of abnormal tissue to exclude malignancy
   d. Intra-oesophageal pH monitor
   e. Bernstein test (acid perfusion of lower oesophagus to reproduce the symptoms of oesophagitis)
   f. Oesophageal manometry

BELSEY MARK IV ANTI-REFLUX OPERATION

Pre-incision
1. General anaesthetic with a double lumen endotracheal tube to allow deflation of the left lung
2. Position – right lateral
3. Skin preparation for left posterolateral thoracotomy

Incision
Left posterolateral thoracotomy via the bed of the 7th rib (see p. 51)

Procedure
(*See* Principles, above)
1. Allow lung to deflate and divide the left pulmonary ligament
2. Divide the pleura overlying the oesophagus below the aortic arch and mobilise the oesophagus. Place a sling around it
3. Ligate and divide the oesophageal branches of the aorta
4. Beware
   a. Opening the opposite pleural space
   b. Damage to the vagi
5. Open the peritoneal sac lying anterior to the thoracic stomach and divide the phreno-oesophageal ligament
6. The stomach and oesophagus are now completely free within the chest
7. Perform the fundoplication in two rows of interrupted sutures around the anterolateral three-quarters of the oesophagus (leaving the posterior quarter of the oesophageal circumference bare)
   a. The first row of sutures buttress the fundus to the oesophagus
   b. The second row of sutures buttress the fundus and oesophagus to the diaphragm
8. Close any residual hiatal deficit with interrupted sutures after the fundoplication has reduced the stomach and lower oesophagus to the abdomen
9. Closure
   a. Drain the haemothorax via an underwater seal drain
   b. Reinflate the left lung and close the thoracotomy (*see* p. 51)

Postoperative management
1. Chest X-ray in recovery
   a. Ensure left lung is fully inflated
   b. Exclude right pneumothorax
2. Commence nasogastric tube feeding on the first postoperative day
3. Remove
   a. Chest drain when the drainage is minimal (2–3 days)
   b. Nasogastric tube at 2–3 days, then continue free fluids until the 6th postoperative day when solids can commence

Complications
1. Early
   a. Right side pneumothorax
   b. Early dysphagia is very common and usually resolves
2. Late
   a. Recurrent gastro-oesophageal reflux (10%)
   b. Stricture at cardia

NISSEN FUNDOPLICATION

Pre-incision
1. General anaesthesia with endotracheal intubation
2. Position – supine
3. Skin preparation for an upper abdominal incision

Incision
Upper midline or laparoscopic approach

Procedure
(*See* Principles, above)
1. Full laparotomy/laparoscopy
2. Retract the left lobe of the liver medially
3. Mobilise the gastric fundus by (Fig. 11)
   a. Ligating and dividing the short gastric vessels
   b. Ligating and dividing the upper branches of the left gastric artery
   c. Divide the peritoneum overlying the oesophagus
4. Beware damage to the spleen
5. Reduce the hiatus hernia if present

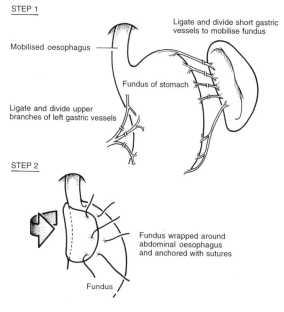

STEP 1

Mobilised oesophagus

Ligate and divide short gastric vessels to mobilise fundus

Fundus of stomach

Ligate and divide upper branches of left gastric vessels

STEP 2

Fundus wrapped around abdominal oesophagus and anchored with sutures

Fundus

Fig. 11   Steps in Nissen fundoplication.

6. Draw the fundus around the posterior oesophagus and perform the fundoplication by suturing its apex loosely to the anterior lower oesophagus and upper body of the stomach with several interrupted non-absorbable sutures
7. Repair any hiatal deficit with several non-absorbable mattress sutures

Closure
1. No drains
2. Close in layers

Postoperative management
Remove the nasogastric tube on the first postoperative day and commence oral fluids

Complications
1. Early
   a. Acute gastric dilatation
   b. Reactionary haemorrhage
   c. Gastric fistula
   d. Dysphagia (usually transient)
2. Late
   Recurrent gastro-oesophageal reflux

ANGELCHIK PROSTHESIS OPERATION
1. Proceed as for a Nissen fundoplication (both open and laparoscopic technique) as far as retraction of the left lobe of the liver (*see* p. 74)
2. Divide the peritoneum lying anteriorly over the lower oesophagus and continue laterally around both sides of the oesophagus until the lowest 2–3 cm of oesophagus is fully mobilised
3. Gently insert the silicone prosthesis around the lower oesophagus and tie the two ties at the free ends together
4. Repair any hiatal deficit with several non-absorbable mattress sutures

Closure and postoperative management
As for Nissen fundoplication (*see* above)

PRINCIPLES OF PEPTIC ULCER SURGERY

Establish the diagnosis
Investigations
1. Endoscopy with biopsy
2. Barium meal
3. Gastric function tests

a. Resting (basal) acid secretion
b. Pentagastrin stimulation test
4. Hormone assay – Gastrin (Zollinger–Ellison)
a. Calcium challenge
b. Secretin challenge

Operation for benign gastric ulcer (including prepyloric ulcers)

	Recurrence (%)	Mortality (%)
Billroth I gastrectomy (including ulcer site)	7	2
Truncal vagotomy, pyloroplasty and excision of ulcer	10	1
Proximal gastric vagotomy and excision of ulcer	10 – GU 30 – PPU	1
Vagotomy and antrectomy (for prepyloric ulcer)	2	2

GU=gastric ulcer; PPU=prepyloric ulcer

Operation for duodenal ulcer (including prepyloric ulcers)

	Recurrence (%)	Mortality (%)
Gastrojejunostomy	40 (including stomal)	1
Billroth II gastrectomy	10 (stomal)	2
Truncal vagotomy and drainage (pyloroplasty, gastroenterostomy)	5–15	1
Proximal gastric vagotomy	5–15	0.05
Truncal vagotomy and antrectomy	2	2

Reasons for recurrent GU
1. Persistence of aetiological factors
   a. Non-steroidal anti-inflammatory drugs
   b. Steroids
2. Misdiagnosed gastric carcinoma
3. Delayed gastric emptying
4. Inadequate gastric resection
5. Duodenogastric reflux

Reasons for recurrent DU (duodenal ulcer) stomal ulcer
1. Inadequate vagotomy

2. Inadequate gastric resection (with retained antrum following Billroth II)
3. Zollinger–Ellison syndrome
   a. G-cell hyperplasia
   b. Pancreatic gastrinoma
4. Hyperparathyroidism

EMERGENCY PEPTIC ULCER SURGERY

Bleeding PU
1. Conservative management
   a. Antacids
   b. H2 antagonist $\Big\}$ Alone, no effect but helpful in combination
2. Endoscopic sclerotherapy
   a. Diathermy cautery
   b. YAG laser

GU
Surgery – Billroth I or II gastrectomy including ulcer site

DU
Surgery – duodenotomy with oversew of bleeding ulcer in combination with definitive procedure for the ulcer (truncal vagotomy and pyloroplasty)

Perforated PU
(See Oversew of a perforated duodenal ulcer, p. 80)
1. GU
   a. Small ulcer – excise the ulcer (to exclude carcinoma of the stomach) and close defect
   b. Large ulcer – partial gastrectomy
2. DU
   Oversew of perforation using an omental patch (with subsequent medical management of acid oversecretion and H. Pyloridi)
3. In all cases full saline peritoneal lavage and a therapeutic course of antibiotics (broad spectrum and metronidazole) commencing before the operation

TRUNCAL VAGOTOMY AND PYLOROPLASTY

Preoperative management
1. Investigations (see principles of peptic ulcer surgery, p. 75)
2. Antibiotics – cephalosporin and metronidazole as the stomach is to be opened. H_2 antagonists result in gastric bacterial colonisation and should be stopped for 48 hours prior to surgery
3. Nasogastric tube
4. IVI

Pre-incision
1. General anaesthetic with endotracheal intubation
2. Position – supine
3. Skin preparation for an upper abdominal incision

Incision
Upper midline

Procedure
1. Full laparotomy (exclude common conditions which mimic peptic ulcer symptoms: gallstones, hiatus hernia)
2. Retract the left lobe of the liver medially to visualise the oesophagus at the hiatus
3. Divide the peritoneum overlying the front of the oesophagus and encircle the abdominal oesophagus with an index finger, dividing the posterior peritoneal oesophageal attachment. Place a sling around the oesophagus
4. Identify, ligate and resect 1–2 cm of
   a. Posterior vagal trunk – lies up to 1 cm distant from posterior right oesophagus in the lesser omentum. Can always be found in the angle of the hiatus
   b. Anterior vagal trunk – lying on the anterior oesophagus
5. Send these specimens for confirmatory histological examination

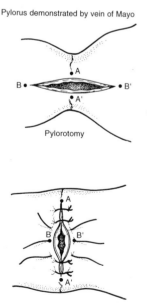

Pylorus demonstrated by vein of Mayo

Pylorotomy

Pyloroplasty closed B to B' using interrupted sutures

Fig. 12 Steps in Heinecke–Mikulicz pyloroplasty.

6. Perform a Heinecke–Mikulicz pyloroplasty (Fig. 12)
   a. Make a longitudinal incision extending equidistant, either side of the pylorus
   b. Close this incision transversely in two layers with interrupted sutures
   c. Closure
      • Haemostasis (especially the spleen)
      • No drains
      • Close in layers

Postoperative management
1. Regular nasogastric aspiration for 24–48 hours until the aspirate is minimal and then commence oral fluids

Investigations
   a. Histological examination of vagal fibres
   b. Hollander insulin test or sham feeding test to confirm complete vagotomy

Complications
1. Early
   a. Leak from pyloroplasty
   b. Acute gastric dilatation (with oedematous pyloroplasty)
   c. Gastric atony
2. Mid – failure of gastric emptying (atony)
3. Late
   a. Diarrhoea
   b. Dumping
   c. Recurrent ulcer

PROXIMAL GASTRIC VAGOTOMY

Proceed as for truncal vagotomy as far as the laparotomy (*see* p. 77)

Procedure
1. Retract the left lobe of the liver medially to expose anterior aspect of the stomach
2. Identify the 'crows foot' of vessels descending onto the pylorus from the lesser omentum. Commence at the most proximal of these vessels, some 8 cm proximal to the pylorus
3. Incise the peritoneum of the lesser omentum and continue this incision proximally up the lesser curve, 1 cm from the junction of lesser omentum and stomach, ligating and dividing all vessels as far as the left gastric vessels
4. Return to the starting point and now ligate and divide all the small vessels lying between the two leaves of the lesser omentum for the length of the incision

5. Now divide the posterior leaf of the lesser omentum, ligating its vessels for the length of this incision
6. Continue the incision at the proximal end of the anterior lesser omentum obliquely upwards to the angle of His, between the fundus and oesophagus, and pass a sling around the oesophagus to retract it
7. Complete the division of the peritoneum from around the cardia and meticulously divide all the longitudinal nerve fibres descending around the oesophagus onto the stomach

Closure
1. Bury the bare area of stomach along the lesser curve by closing the gastric serosa over the two layers of lesser omental peritoneum with a continuous suture to reduce the risks of gastric perforation due to ischaemia
2. No drain
3. Close in layers

Postoperative management
Commence oral fluids the next day

Complications
1. Early – acute lesser curve necrosis
2. Late – recurrent ulcer 5–10%

OVERSEW OF A PERFORATED DUODENAL ULCER
1. Establish the diagnosis
    a. Clinically
    b. Free gas on abdominal X-rays (80%)
    c. Leucocytosis
    d. Raised amylase (300–1000 units)
2. Resuscitation
    a. IVI – Restore blood pressure with colloid and, if anaemic, transfuse peroperatively
    b. Catheterise to monitor urine output
3. Antibiotics
    a. Broad spectrum and metronidazole for a full therapeutic course commencing at the suspicion of the diagnosis
    b. Analgesia for peritonitis
4. Uncertain diagnosis
5. Exclude
    a. Myocardial infarction
    b. Leaking aorta aneurysm
    c. Acute pancreatitis
    d. Acute cholecystitis

Pre-incision
1. General anaesthetic with endotracheal intubation
2. Position – supine
3. Skin preparation of the whole of the abdomen but with the towels placed for an upper abdominal incision

Incision
Upper midline or laparoscopically

Procedure
1. On entering the peritoneum, there is a rush of free gas, swab the intra-peritoneal fluid for microbiological examination and suck out this fluid, wipe out any large deposits of food or debris
2. Identify the perforation and excise the free edge of the ulcer
3. If the ulcer is small, then close transversely with interrupted absorbable sutures. Cover the repair with free greater omentum and suture in place with non-absorbable sutures
4. If the ulcer is large, then closing the defect may result in pyloric stenosis, so plug with free greater omentum and suture in place with non-absorbable sutures
5. Full peritoneal lavage with warm saline

Controversies
1. Use of an antiseptic (e.g. noxythiolin) or an antibiotic (e.g. tetracycline) in saline lavage
2. Drainage of the wound closure, or potential abscess cavities (subphrenic spaces, subhepatic spaces, pelvis)

Closure
1. Haemostasis
2. Swabs and instruments
3. Close in layers

Postoperative management
1. Commence antacid therapy (H_2 antagonists) immediately post-surgery as no definitive surgery has been undertaken for the ulcer
2. Continue nasogastric aspiration until minimal
3. Commence oral fluids when bowel sounds return, nasogastric aspirate is minimal and flatus is passed per rectum

Complications
1. Early
   a. Bleeding
      • From ulcer edge
      • From co-existent posterior ulcer
   b. Pyloric stenosis with oedema
   c. Ileus

d. Peritonitis
e. Abscess
  • Subphrenic
  • Subhepatic
  • Pelvic
2. Late
  a. Recurrent ulceration (70% if no definitive ulcer procedure has been undertaken)
  b. Obstruction from post-peritonitis adhesions

GASTRECTOMY (BILLROTH I, BILLROTH II, TOTAL)

Indications
1. Benign gastric ulcer
  a. Chronic, not responding to medical treatment
  b. Complicated
    • Bleeding
    • Perforated
    • Pyloric stenosis
2. Carcinoma of the stomach

Preoperative management
1. Investigations
  a. Elective surgery
    • Haemoglobin and correct anaemia if present
    • Endoscopy and biopsy
    • Barium meal
    • Benign ulcer – gastric secretion test
    • Malignant ulcer, exclude metastases – liver function tests
    • Liver ultrasound
    • Liver isotope scan
  b. Emergency surgery
    Bleeding ulcer
      • Endoscopy
      • Transfuse
      • Monitor CVP
    Perforation
      • Plain X-rays (free gas)
      • Amylase
2. Tubes
  a. IVI
  b. Nasogastric tube
  c. Catheter
  d. CVP line for emergency surgery
3. Antibiotics
  Broad spectrum with metronidazole

Pre-incision
1. General anaesthesia with endotracheal intubation
2. Position – supine
3. Skin preparation – prepare and towel up for an upper abdominal incision

Incision
1. Upper midline
2. Alternatives
   a. Upper transverse
   b. Left upper paramedian
   c. Thoracoabdominal for total gastrectomy

BILLROTH I GASTRECTOMY (Fig. 13)
Indications
1. Benign gastric ulcer
2. Small prepyloric carcinoma
3. Acquired pyloric stenosis

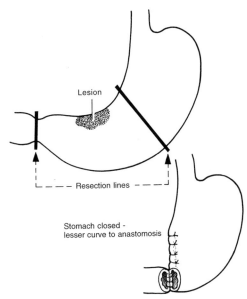

Fig. 13 Steps in Billroth I gastrectomy.

Procedure
1. Full laparotomy
2. Open the gastrocolic omentum, divide and ligate the right gastroepiploic vessels and the distal gastric branches of the left gastroepiploic vessels
3. Ligate and divide the right gastric vessels
4. Divide the lesser omentum, ligate and divide the lower branches of the left gastric artery and vein
5. Kocherise the duodenum and mobilise the first part of the duodenum
6. Place a soft bowel clamp across the first part of the duodenum and a crushing clamp across the pylorus
7. Place a soft clamp across the width of the mid body of the stomach, including any pathology with the distal specimen. Place a crushing clamp parallel and distal to this and excise the distal stomach within the crushing clamps
8. Close the gastric remnant in two layers from the lesser curve for about two-thirds of the width of the stomach
9. Anastomose the gastric orifice to the first part of the duodenum in two layers

BILLROTH II (POLYA) GASTRECTOMY

Indications
As for Billroth I

Procedure
1. Perform gastectomy as for Billroth I as far as the removal of the specimen
2. Close the duodenal stump in two layers
3. Locate the duodenojejunal flexure and bring up the most available proximal loop of jejunum. Place a soft clamp transversely to isolate the anti-mesenteric border of 10 cm of jejunum
4. Close the gastric remnant in two layers from the lesser curve for about half of the width of the stomach
5. Anastomose the gastric remnant in two layers to the anti-mesenteric border of the jejunal loop

(Arguments for retrocolic versus antecolic gastrojejunostomy are probably spurious)

TOTAL GASTRECTOMY

Indications
Malignant gastric tumour

Procedure
1. Proceed as for Billroth I gastrectomy, divide the right and left gastrocolic vessels and the right gastric vessels
2. Divide the left gastric vessels
3. Divide the short gastric vessels individually
4. Beware
   a. Spleen
   b. Tail of pancreas
5. Place soft bowel clamps across the first part of the duodenum and oesophagus with crushing clamps on the adjacent stomach. Excise and remove the gastric specimen
6. Close the duodenal stump in two layers
7. Fashion a Roux loop of 60 cm from proximal jejunum and anastomose this to the distal oesophagus
8. Closure
   a. Drain all anastomoses and duodenal stump
   b. Place a nasogastric tube
   c. Close in layers

Postoperative management
1. Investigations
   a. Check haemoglobin and transfuse accordingly
   b. Histology of specimen
2. Remove
   a. Nasogastric tube when the aspirate is minimal
   b. Drains when drainage is minimal but leave the duodenal stump drain for 5 days (thus reducing the morbidity of a duodenal fistula)
3. Commence oral fluids with the passage of flatus per rectum

Complications
1. Early
   a. Gastric outflow obstruction at anastomosis
      • Oedema
      • Stricture
   b. Duodenal stump leakage with Billroth II
2. Late
   a. Dumping
      • 90% early dumping
      • 10% late dumping
   b. Nutritional
      • Iron deficiency
      • B_{12} deficiency
      • Calcium deficiency
   c. Weight loss
   d. Increased incidence of reactivation of tuberculosis
   e. Bilious vomiting with Billroth II gastrectomy
   f. Diarrhoea

g. Increased incidence of gallstones
h. Increased incidence of carcinoma of the stomach

RAMSTEDT'S OPERATION FOR PYLORIC STENOSIS

Preoperative management
1. Establish the diagnosis
   a. Clinical examination
   b. Test feed
   c. Barium meal
2. Correct
   a. Dehydration
   b. Metabolic alkalosis
   c. Hypokalaemia
3. Gastric lavage via a nasogastric tube
4. Nasogastric tube
5. IVI

Pre-incision
1. Operating theatre temperature >17°C to reduce chilling
2. General anaesthesia with endotracheal intubation
3. Position – supine and otherwise well wrapped
4. Skin preparation for an upper abdominal incision

Incision
Upper right transverse (over the palpable pyloric tumour) muscle splitting

Procedure
1. Deliver the pyloric tumour into the incision
2. Pyloromyotomy – incise the peritoneum over the length of the tumour and split both the longitudinal and circular muscle fibres down to the submucosa
3. Beware
   a. Opening the duodenal mucosa, suspected if any bubbles of gastric juice and air appear within the incision
   b. If so, repair with a fine absorbable suture

Closure
No drains
Close in layers

Postoperative management
Test feed the baby on small amounts of milk 4 hours after waking up and gradually increase over 48 hours
Persistent vomiting – stop the feeds and recommence slowly 8 hours later

Complications
Early
    a. Peritonitis due to unrecognised mucosal
       perforation
    b. Inadequate pyloromyotomy with persistent
       vomiting
Late
Recurrent pyloric stenosis is rare

LAPAROTOMY FOR BOWEL OBSTRUCTION

Preoperative management
1. Resuscitate
   Rehydrate and correct electrolyte losses (sodium and
   potassium)
2. Investigations
    a. Electrolytes
    b. Full blood count/PCV to assess dehydration
      • ? Anaemia
      • ? leucocytosis with strangulation
    c. ECG
      • Effects of electrolyte disturbances
    d. AXR
      • Level of obstruction
      • Fluid levels on erect film
      • Free gas with concomitant perforation
    e. Small bowel enema/follow through
    f. NG tube
      • Empty the stomach prior to anaesthesia
    g. IVI
    h. Catheterise
3. Broad spectrum and metronidazole antibiotic prophylaxis

Indications for surgery
1. Simple obstruction not relieved by conservative measures after
   24–48 hours
2. Evidence of
    a. Peritonism (pyrexia)
    b. Strangulated bowel (leucocytosis)
3. Free gas on plain X-rays

Pre-incision
1. General anaesthesia and endotracheal intubation
2. Position – supine
3. Skin preparation of all of abdomen, nipples to thighs

Incision
Right paramedian at the level of the umbilicus

Procedure
1. Open the peritoneum carefully: beware underlying distended bowel
2. Suck out free fluid, sending a specimen for microbiological examination

Small bowel obstruction
1. Commence in right iliac fossa, looking for collapsed distal ileum
2. Trace the bowel proximally from this as far as the agent of obstruction (adhesions, intra-abdominal hernia, tumour)
3. Relieve obstruction

MANAGEMENT OF JUVENILE INTUSSUSCEPTION

Diagnosis
1. Clinical picture of a 2–3 month old infant that is white with pain, screaming and passing red currant jelly stools is not typical
2. Age range from a few days to 4–6 years old
3. Symptoms may last for a few minutes each hour, otherwise the child may be asymptomatic
4. The 'tumour' may be impalpable if it lies under a costal margin
5. Therefore the diagnosis is one of clinical suspicion, *and a barium enema is mandatory*

Hydrostatic reduction
1. A child with early symptoms can undergo a barium enema, a child with 24 hours + of symptoms ought to undergo attempted radiological reduction using a water soluble contrast in case of colonic perforation
2. If there is any doubt at all about peritonism (particularly with a long history) then proceed directly to surgery
3. Hydrostatic reduction (if mechanically possible) can be achieved with a pressure of a column of barium 1 m high. If that fails consider early surgery

Surgery
1. General anaesthesia
2. Broad spectrum and metronidazole antibiotic cover
3. Prep the whole abdomen
4. Right side transverse incision
5. Locate the intussusception and *gently reduce by pushing the intussusceptum out of the intussuscipiens.* Never reduce by traction.
6. Once reduced check the viability of the bowel
7. If there is any doubt about bowel viability or the pathological aetiology of the intussusception then resect the suspicious bowel

Hepatobiliary surgery

PRINCIPLES OF CHOLECYSTECTOMY

Indications

1. Calculous cholecystitis
2. (Typhoid carrier)
3. (Carcinoma of the gall bladder – rarely, an early cancer is found incidentally within a gallbladder removed for cholelithiasis)

Preoperative management

1. Investigations
   a. Ultrasound of gallbladder and bile ducts
   b. Cholecystogram
   c. If previously jaundiced
      • Liver function tests
      • HBS Ag status
      • Clotting screen
   d. History of allergic reaction to X-ray contrast media
   e. PTC/ERCP if jaundiced
2. The mortality of cholecystectomy in cirrhosis/portal hypertension is up to 10%
3. Vitamin K if recently jaundiced
4. Antibiotics
   a. Broad spectrum now generally accepted as one dose or three dose prophylaxis
   b. Risk groups for infection in bilary surgery
      • >70 years old
      • Diabetic
      • On steroids
      • Jaundiced or recently jaundiced
      • Common bile duct exploration
      • Malignancy involving the biliary tree
      • Common bile duct stones or stricture
5. IVI (with prehydration or 10% mannitol infusion if jaundiced)
6. Nasogastric tube to deflate the stomach peroperatively

Pre-incision

1. General anaesthetic (avoiding hepatotoxic agents such as halothane) and endotracheal intubation
2. Position – supine on an X-ray operating table
3. Skin preparation for an upper abdominal incision
4. Empty bladder prior to laparoscopic procedure

Incision

1. Kochers right subcostal
2. Right paramedian   } All equally acceptable
3. Right upper transverse
4. Laparoscopic with port sites at the umbilicus, midline epigastrium and right subcostal in the mid-clavicular line

Procedure

1. Full laparotomy/laparoscopy with particular attention to
   a. 'Saints Triad'
      - Gallstones
      - Hiatus hernia
      - Sigmoid diverticular disease
   b. Other causes of upper abdominal pain
      - Peptic ulcer
      - Carcinoma of the stomach
      - Pancreatic carcinoma
      - Chronic pancreatitis

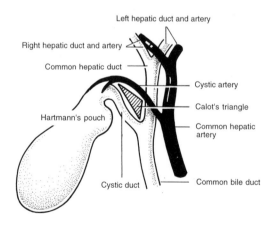

Fig. 14   Surgery anatomy of gallbladder.

2. Open cholecystectomy
   a. Display the gall bladder
      • Pack off the small bowel
      • Retract the stomach and duodenum downwards
      • Retract the liver upwards
   b. Retract the gall bladder laterally, held in a sponge holder or Moynihan gall bladder clamp and incise the peritoneum over the right free border of the lesser omentum
3. Laparoscopic cholecystectomy
   Grasp and retract the gallbladder fundus in a lateral direction
4. Dissect out Calot's triangle bordered by (Fig. 14)
   a. Cystic duct inferiorly
   b. Cystic artery superiorly
   c. Common hepatic and right hepatic duct on the left
   Before any structure is divided it is absolutely essential to identify the cystic duct and artery, and be absolutely certain of the position of the structures of the right free border of the lesser omentum (common bile duct and common hepatic duct, hepatic artery and portal vein) (Fig. 15)
5. Ligate/clip and divide the cystic artery in continuity
6. Cannulate the cystic duct and aspirate bile for microbiological examination
7. Perform the operative cholangiogram
   a. Remove all instruments and radio-opaque swabs
   b. Tilt the operating table 10° to the right (so the bile ducts do not overlie the spine)

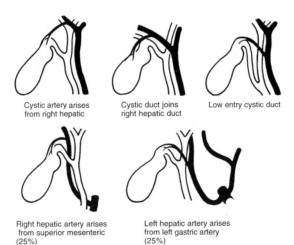

Cystic artery arises from right hepatic

Cystic duct joins right hepatic duct

Low entry cystic duct

Right hepatic artery arises from superior mesenteric (25%)

Left hepatic artery arises from left gastric artery (25%)

Fig. 15 Common anatomical variants.

   c. Stop the ventilator during X-ray exposure

   d. Take at least two films, after the injection of 2 and 10 ml of contrast

8. Points to establish on the operative cholangiogram
    a. Clear visualisation of all the common bile and hepatic ducts with delineation of the anatomy
    b. No filling defects or strictures
    c. Free flow into the duodenum in all films
    d. Common bile duct not dilated greater than 11 mm
    e. Minimal retrograde flow of contrast into the pancreatic ducts

9. If all these are established then withdraw the catheter and proceed

10. Problems with peroperative cholangiography
    a. Introduction of air bubbles, mimicking radiolucent stones
    b. Spasm of the sphincter of Oddi
    c. Contrast in the duodenum obscuring the terminal common bile duct and ampulla

11. Complete the cholecystectomy
    a. Transfix and ligate/clip the cystic duct within 1 cm of the common bile duct with an absorbable suture or metal clip
    b. Divide the peritoneal reflection between the gallbladder and the liver and dissect the gallbladder out of its hepatic bed. Remove the gallbladder at this stage in an open procedure
    c. Use diathermy coagulation to control bleeding from the liver bed
    d. Remove the gallbladder via the umbilical port site if undertaking a laparoscopic procedure

12. Examine the gallbladder and gallstones. Send the gallbladder for histological examination to exclude co-existing malignancy. Swab the gallbladder mucosa and send for microbiological culture and sensitivity. Any postoperative wound infection will be due to bile contamination.

13. Closure
    a. Absolute haemostasis
       • Cystic artery
       • Gallbladder bed
    b. Suction drain to gallbladder bed
    c. If an open cholecystectomy leads to exploration of the common bile duct then bring the T-tube out by a separate stab incision
    d. Close in layers

Postoperative management

1. Accurate measurements of drainage essential; suspect a significant leak if >300 ml of bile is drained daily from the suction drain to the gallbladder bed during the first 24 postoperative hours

2. Investigations
   a. Histology of gallbladder
   b. If T-tube present – T-tube cholangiogram to establish normal biliary flow and exclude retained stones prior to its removal

Complications
1. Early
   a. Biliary leak
   b. Ileus
   c. Wound infection
   d. Persistent jaundice with a retained stone
   e. Septicaemia
   f. Pancreatitis
2. Late
   a. Cholangitis – retained stone
   b. Biliary stricture

EXPLORATION OF THE COMMON BILE DUCT

Indications for choledochotomy/choledochoscopy

Abnormality noted on a preoperative or peroperative cholangiogram
Obstructive jaundice not due to pancreatic or ampullary disease
Palpable stones in the bile ducts

Factors in considering methods of choledochotomy

	Mortality (%)
Cholecystectomy	<1
Supraduodenal choledochotomy	<2
Transduodenal choledochotomy	<4

Supraduodenal choledochotomy
   a. Place two stay sutures either side of the proposed 2 cm longitudinal incision in the common bile duct in the right free border of the lesser omentum
   b. Kocherise the duodenum to expose the full length of the common bile duct
   c. Incise the common bile duct longitudinally
   d. Close the choledochotomy with an absorbable suture over a latex T-tube brought out through a tunnel of greater omentum

Closure and postoperative management
As for cholecystectomy (*see* p. 89)

SPLENECTOMY

Indications
1. Trauma, if splenic preservation impractical (beware associated left kidney injury)
2. Haematological
   a. Haemolytic anaemia
   b. Myelofibrosis
   c. Leukaemia
3. Not now commonly part of the staging of lymphoma
4. Part of surgery for portal hypertension and pancreatic resection

Preoperative management
1. Trauma
   a. Resuscitate
      • Test urine for haematuria
      • Plain X-ray may show fractures of overlying ribs
      • Peritoneal lavage
      • Abdominal ultrasound may show splenic fracture and free fluid
   b. Catheterise
   c. Nasogastric tube
   d. IVI
2. Haematological
   Check
   a. Haemoglobin
   b. White cell count – transfuse accordingly
   c. Platelet count
      Give pneumococcal vaccine 2 weeks prior to elective surgery
3. Antibiotics
   In all cases broad spectrum and metronidazole
4. Portal hypertension

Pre-incision
1. General anaesthetic with endotracheal intubation
2. Position – supine
3. Skin preparation for an upper abdominal incision

Incision
1. Left paramedian in trauma (better access to the rest of the abdomen) or
2. Left Kocher subcostal

Procedure
1. Trauma – suck out all free blood and clots
2. Place the left hand on the spleen and draw it down to divide the lieno renal ligament lying posteriorly
3. Now deliver the spleen to the abdominal incision

4. Examine the spleen – in trauma consider splenic repair and preservation
5. Ligate and divide
   a. Short gastric vessels
   b. Left gastro-epiploic vessel
   (Bury the stumps of these vessels on the greater curve of the stomach with an absorbable serosal suture to minimise the subsequent risk of ischaemic gastric perforation due to a ligature placed directly on the stomach)
6. Gently separate the tail of the pancreas from the splenic vessels
7. Clamp, separately divide and doubly ligate the splenic artery and splenic vein
8. Beware
   a. Tail of pancreas
   b. Splenic flexure of colon
   c. Left kidney and adrenal
9. Complete splenectomy by dividing the residual peritoneal attachments to the stomach and colon
10. Complete the laparotomy (*see* Laparotomy for abdominal trauma, p. 197)

Closure
1. Meticulous haemostasis
2. Peritoneal saline lavage
3. Trauma – place a suction drain to the tail of the pancreas
4. Close in layers

Postoperative management
1. Remove
   a. Nasogastric tube when aspirate is minimal (24–48 hours)
   b. Drain when drainage is minimal (24–48 hours)
2. Commence
   a. Oral fluids when flatus passed per rectum
   b. Long term pencillin V – 250 mg daily (to reduce the risk of opportunist infection, especially pneumococcus)
   c. Course of pneumococcal vaccine
3. Trauma
   Give pneumococcal vaccine during immediate postoperative period
4. Long term penicillin for children, associated immunodeficiency, and to cover potentially infective procedures (e.g. dental surgery)

Complications
1. Early
   a. Acute gastric dilatation

   b. Fundal ischaemia
      • Gastric perforation
      • Haematemesis
   c. Pancreatic fistula
   d. Portal vein thrombosis
   e. Reactionary haemorrhage from splenic vessels
2. Late
   a. Increased infection
      • Pneumococcal
      • Viral
   b. Thrombocytosis

INTERNAL DRAINAGE OF A PANCREATIC PSEUDOCYST

Indications – pseudocyst
1. >5 cm in diameter
2. Symptomatic
3. Infection

Preoperative management
1. Investigations
   a. Ultrasound
   b. Barium meal
   c. CT
   d. ERCP
2. Antibiotics
   a. Broad spectrum
   b. Metronidazole
   3. Nasogastric tube
   4. IVI

Pre-incision
1. General anaesthetic with endotracheal intubation
2. Position – supine on an X-ray table
3. Skin preparation for an upper abdominal incision

Incision
Upper midline

Procedure
1. Full laparotomy
2. Insert a wide bore needle via the lesser or greater omentum into the cyst and aspirate cyst contents for
   a. Microbiological examination
   b. Cytological examination
   c. Amylase estimation
3. Peroperative cystography can be performed by injecting 20 ml of Hypaque into the cyst cavity

4. Perform an anterior longitudinal gastrotomy of about 8 cm in length. Achieve haemostasis at the gastric edges
5. Make a 5–6 cm linear incision in the posterior wall of the stomach to enter the pseudocyst
6. Suck out the fluid and remove any solid debris
7. Oversew the edges of the cyst gastrotomy with an absorbable suture
8. Close the anterior gastrotomy in two layers

Closure
1. No drains
2. Close in layers

Alternative methods of drainage
1. Cyst lying adjacent to head of pancreas – cystduodenostomy
2. Cyst lying in transverse mesocolon – cyst-jejunostomy Roux-en-Y
3. Cyst lying at the tail of the pancreas – resect

Postoperative management
1. Remove nasogastric tube when aspirate is minimal
2. Commence oral fluids when flatus is passed per rectum
3. Investigation repeat ultrasound/CT

Complications
1. Early
   a, Secondary haemorrhage from vessels of the cyst wall
   b. Recurrent cyst
   c. Fistula from anastomotic leak
2. Late
   Recurrent cyst

'TRIPLE BYPASS' OPERATION FOR CARCINOMA OF THE HEAD OF THE PANCREAS

Preoperative management
1. Investigations
   a. Diagnostic
      • Liver function tests
      • Ultrasound of biliary tree and pancreas
      • Percutaneous transhepatic cholangiogram
      • ERCP with pancreatic cytology
      • CT
   b. Therapeutic – clotting screen; if the prothrombin time is abnormal then give parenteral Vitamin K
   c. Preoperative percutaneous biliary decompression has not been shown to improve operative mortality and morbidity, and carries a significant morbidity

2. Antibiotics – broad spectrum and metronidazole
3. IVI with either prehydration or 10% mannitol infusion peroperatively to protect the renal tubules by osmotic diuresis
4. Catheterise
5. Nasogastric tube

Pre-incision
1. General anaesthesia with endotracheal intubation
2. Position – supine on X-ray table (if percutaneous cholangiography is required)
3. Skin preparation for an upper abdominal incision

Incision
Upper midline

Procedure
1. Full laparotomy
   a. Assess the resectability of the tumour
   b. Evidence of metastases (liver, pre-aortic nodes, peritoneum)
   c. Tumour size and fixation
2. If the tumour is considered to be unresectable then proceed to a palliative bypass procedure after biopsying the tumour

Method of biopsy
1. Trucut needle
   a. Transduodenally
   b. Direct
2. Open
   a. Pancreas
   b. Regional nodes

Cholecystojejunostomy
1. Decompress the distended tense gallbladder by fashioning a fundal purse-string suture and inserting a gallbladder trochar and suction cannula through a cholecystostomy within the purse-string
2. Cholangiography may be performed at this stage, if the cystic duct enters the common bile duct close to the tumour, then consider anastomosing the common hepatic duct to a Roux loop of jejunum (hepatico-jejunostomy)
3. Anastomose the gallbladder fundus in two layers to an available loop of proximal jejunum

Gastroenterostomy
Anastomose the stomach side-to-side to a loop of jejunum proximal to the cholecyst-jejunostomy

Entero-enterostomy
Anastomose a segment of jejunum between the gastrojejunostomy and the cholecyst-jejunostomy side-to-side to a segment of jejunum distal to the cholecyst-jejunostomy in two layers

Purpose of bypass procedures
1. Gastro-jejunostomy
   Bypasses duodenal obstruction by the pancreatic tumour
2. Cholecyst-jejunostomy/hepatico-jejunostomy
   Maintains biliary drainage (unless the tumour invades as far as the cystic duct which may enter the common bile duct low down)
3. Entero-enterostomy
   Diverts small bowel content away from the cholecyst-jejunostomy reducing the risk of cholangitis

Closure
1. Meticulous haemostasis in the jaundiced patient
2. Drain anastomoses
3. Close in layers

Postoperative management
1. Aspirate nasogastric tube until the aspirate is minimal and commence oral fluids at the passage of flatus per rectum
2. Investigations
   a. Histology of tumour
   b. Liver function tests
   c. Renal function

Complications
1. Early
   a. Septicaemia
   b. Cholangitis
   c. Ileus
   d. Obstruction of anastomoses with oedema
2. Late
   a. Recurrent jaundice – 20%
   b. Cholangitis
   c. Tumour spread
   d. Gastric outflow obstruction with tumour spread – 15%

PRINCIPLES OF PANCREATICO–DUODENECTOMY

Indications
1. Potentially resectable tumour of pancreatic head
2. Low cholangiocarcinoma
3. Ampullary or duodenal carcinoma
4. Chronic pancreatitis for pain relief

Preoperative management
Pre-incision and incision, as for 'Triple bypass' for carcinoma of the head of pancreas (see p. 97)

Procedure
1. Full laparotomy, exclude any evidence of disseminated disease (nodes, peritoneal seedlings, liver metastases)
2. Kocherise the duodenum, lifting the pancreatic head with the portal vein off the retroperitoneal structures (including the IVC) and continuing to the left until the left renal vein is fully exposed
3. Open the peritoneum overlying the root of the mesentery as it emerges from under the pancreatic neck and gently explore the recess between the superior mesenteric artery and vein and the neck of the pancreas lying anteriorly
4. Do not proceed if the tumour has invaded either of these vascular structures, continue as with the 'Triple bypass' procedure (see p. 97)
5. If there is a plane of dissection between these vessels and the pancreatic neck, then the tumour is resectable: divide the small veins entering the superior mesenteric/portal vein from the pancreas, ligate and divide the gastroduodenal and inferior pancreatico-duodenal arteries
6. Divide the neck of the pancreas, the proximal jejunum, distal stomach and common bile duct, remove the specimen (Fig. 16)

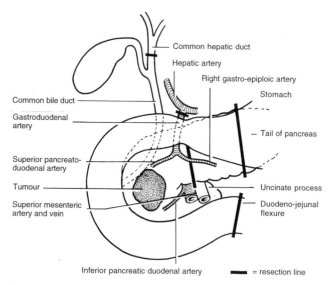

Fig. 16 Anatomy of pancreatico-duodenectomy.

7. Anastomose the proximal jejunum first to the body of the pancreas over a stent (e.g. umbilical catheter)
8. Now anastomose this loop of jejunum to the gastric remnant and then the common bile duct over a T-tube

Closure
1. Place non-suction drains around pancreatic anastomosis
2. Attention to meticulous haemostasis
3. Close in layers

Postoperative management
1. Histology and resection margins of tumour
2. T-tube cholangiogram prior to removal of T-tube
3. Keep pancreatic stent in place until eating normally, afebrile and minimal drainage from the pancreatic drains

Complications
1. Early
   a. Pancreatic fistula, keep nil by mouth and administer somatostatin to reduce pancreatic secretion
   b. Haemorrhage, including increased risk of upper GI bleeding
2. Late
   a. Recurrent cancer
   b. Exocrine pancreatic failure with stricture of pancreatic anastomosis
   c. Cholangitis due to stricture of choledocho-jejunostomy

PRINCIPLES OF HEPATIC RESECTION

Indications
1. Hepatic tumour
   a. Benign
      • 'Pill' tumour
      • Adenoma
      • Symptomatic focal nodular hyperplasia
   b. Malignant – Primary
      • Hepatoblastoma
      • Hepatocellular
      • Secondary carcinoma (see Table below)
2. Hepatic cyst
   a. Congenital – leave
   b. Hydatid – only treat if symptomatic
3. Trauma
   a. 80% of serious liver injuries have concomitant serious injury to other viscera (*see* Laparotomy for abdominal trauma, p. 197)
   b. Liver + duodenum/pancreas – 50%
   c. Liver + colon – 20%

Place of surgery in the management of hepatic secondaries
Resection surgery is worthwhile for
1. Colorectal primary (up to three unilobar metastases with 25% 5-year survival)
2. Symptomatic carcinoid (consider embolisation)
3. Others; Wilms, renal adenocarcinoma

Liver metastasis from colorectal primary

	Mean survival, months (no treatment)	Mean survival, months (hepatic resection)	5 year survival, (%)
Stage 1 – solitary metastasis	16	24	30
Stage 2 – cluster of metastases	10	17	20
Stage 3 – scattered metastases	6	not applicable	

Hepatic artery embolisation/ligation for endocrine secreting liver metastases
1. Never in the presence of jaundice
2. Needs preoperative angiography
   a. Show pathology
   b. Show anatomy
3. Infuse dextrose 10% and insulin during the procedure to protect hepatocytes
4. Needs 48 hours of parenteral antibiotic prophylaxis
5. Best results in carcinoid

Investigation in hepatic malignancy
1. Liver function tests
2. 5 gamma glutamyl transferase
3. Alphafetoprotein
4. Gut hormone screen
5. Liver ultrasound
6. Hepatic artery and portal vein angiography
7. Inferior vena cavagram
8. CT/MRI
9. Biopsy
   a. Fine needle aspiration ⎫
   b. True cut biopsy   ⎬ May seed tumour
   c. Laparoscopic   ⎭

Anatomical and physiological factors
1. The 'surgical' right and left lobes of the liver are determined by the vascular anatomy of the portal veins and hepatic artery

2. The right lobe of the liver lies to the right of a line that follows the gallbladder fossa and passes back to the IVC (Fig. 17)

Postoperative recovery
Following hemihepatectomy in a non-cirrhotic liver, compensatory regeneration is usually complete in 3–6 months

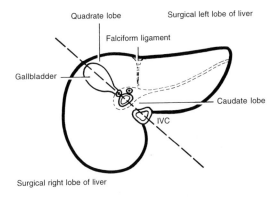

Fig. 17 CT scan view of liver to demonstrate the surgical right and left nodes.

Colorectal surgery

PRINCIPLES OF BOWEL PREPARATION FOR COLORECTAL SURGERY

1. Never on totally obstructed bowel
2. Only with great care from above on partially obstructed bowel with assistance of enemata
3. All need broad spectrum and metronidazole antibiotic prophylaxis

Traditional (and very old-fashioned)

1. Commence on the 5th preoperative day – oral magnesium sulphate and a disposable enema
2. 4th and 3rd preoperative day – low residue diet and magnesium sulphate with daily soap and water enemata
3. 2nd and last preoperative day – fluid diet and castor oil with daily soap and water enemata
4. Comment
   a. Requires admission 5–6 days before surgery
   b. Cleanliness of bowel mucosa not as good as the laxative method and whole gut irrigation
   c. Relatively safe in partial obstruction

Laxative method

1. Commence on the day before surgery
2. Give 75–150 g Mannitol in 300–1000 ml of water orally or 1–2 sachets of Picolax or Kleenprep and two high enemata on the day before surgery
3. Comment
   a. Bowel cleanliness not as good as the whole gut irrigation method
   b. May produce considerable gaseous distension

Whole gut irrigation

1. Commence on the day before surgery
2. Give an oral premed of
   a. Metoclopramide 10 mg

   b. Diazepam 15 mg
   c. Magnesium sulphate 5 mg
3. Pass a soft nasogastric tube as far as the duodenum under X-ray control
4. Irrigate with normal saline (at body temperature, 37°C) at 2–4 l per hour until the anal effluent runs crystal clear
5. Comment
   a. Gives the cleanest bowel preparation
   b. May cause severe water and electrolyte imbalance, especially in the elderly
6. Therefore, needs electrolyte check before and after the procedure; beware congestive cardiac failure with fluid overload and avoid in poor myocardial state

Bowel preparation for emergency colonic surgery
1. Irrigation from below prior to surgery
2. Irrigate the colon on the table via a caecostomy tube

APPENDICECTOMY

Preoperative management
1. Investigations
   a. White cell count
   b. Urinalysis, exclude UTI
   c. Ultrasound
2. If dehydrated due to vomiting, then rehydrate with saline
3. Antibiotic prophylaxis
   a. Metronidazole by suppository
   b. Evidence of perforation – add parenteral broad spectrum antibiotic

Pre-incision
1. General anaesthesia and endotracheal intubation
2. Position – supine
3. Skin preparation for an incision in the right iliac fossa, but prepare all the abdomen

Incision
Grid iron (right iliac fossa over MacBurney's point, two thirds of the way between the umbilicus and the anterior superior iliac spine)

Procedure
1. Deepen the incision by splitting the muscle layers in the line of their fibres
2. As the peritoneum is opened, remove a sample of peritoneal fluid for microbiological examination
3. Withdraw the caecum gently, locate and deliver the appendix

4. Place haemostatic forceps across the appendix mesentery and divide it, ligating the vessels
5. Place a purse-string suture around the taenia coli, 2 cm from the base of the appendix
6. Place crushing forceps just distal to the base of the appendix and ligate the base of the appendix with an absorbable ligature just proximal to this clip
7. Remove the appendix flush with the caecal side of the crushing forceps. Send for histological examination
8. Invaginate the appendix stump in the caecum and tie the purse-string to bury the stump
9. Perform a local peritoneal toilet

Problem
1. Not appendicitis, exclude
   a. Mesenteric adenitis
   b. Right tubo-ovarian pathology
   c. Cholecystitis
   d. Ileitis
      • Yersinia
      • Crohn's
   e. Carcinoma of the caecum
2. Incidental Meckel's diverticulum
   a. Normal – leave
   b. Inflamed – remove
3. Appendicitis in the presence of Crohn's disease
   a. Ileal Crohn's – perform appendicectomy
   b. Caecal Crohn's – leave appendix and drain the peritoneum

Closure
1. Close in layers
2. No drains
3. If the wound is severely contaminated then irrigate with antiseptic solution

Postoperative management
1. Investigate histology of appendix
2. Rare problems
   a. Appendix carcinoid – no further treatment necessary
   b. Adenocarcinoma – needs a right hemicolectomy
3. Microbiological results from peritoneal fluid
4. Continue metronidazole suppositories for 48 hours

Complications
1. Early
   a. Infection
      • Peritonitis
      • Septicaemia

- Wound
- Abscess – pelvic
- Subphrenic
  b. Ileus
  c. Haemorrhage from appendix mesentery (usually reactionary)
  d. Portal pyaemia
  e. Fistula
2. Late
  Adhesions
  - Small bowel obstruction
  - Fallopian tube obstruction

ILEOSTOMY

Indications
1. Total colectomy
2. Defunctioning
   a. To protect ileo-anal anastomosis
   b. Severe colitis

Preoperative management
1. Examine the patient standing, sitting and lying flat to determine the appropriate site in the right iliac fossa for the stoma. Never in a skin fold or near a scar. Introduce the patient to the stoma therapist and encourage psychological support
2. Investigations – those appropriate to the pathology
   a. Ulcerative colitis
   b. Toxic megacolon
   c. Familial polyposis coli
3. IVI
4. Catheter   ⎫
5. Nasogastric tube ⎬ For total colectomy
6. Broad spectrum and metronidazole antibiotic prophylaxis

Pre-incision
1. General anaesthetic with endotracheal intubation
2. Position
   a. Lithotomy – Trendelenberg with Lloyd Davis stirrups for panproctocolectomy
   b. Supine for total colectomy with rectal preservation
3. Skin preparation of all of abdomen including perineum for panproctocolectomy

Incision
Left paramedian

Procedure

1. After the colon ± rectum have been mobilised and resected, usually with the last 10–20 cm of terminal ileum, divide the mesentery preserving all branches proximal to the terminal ileocolic vessels and examine the cut end of ileum to ensure bleeding and viability
2. Cut out a 3 cm disc of skin at the designated ileostomy site, and a further disc of all layers deep to this including the peritoneum
3. Pass the ileal end through the ileostomy hole to protrude by 5 cm and close the lateral space between mesentery and parietal peritoneum with a continuous absorbable suture

Alternative – extraperitoneal method

1. Do not open the peritoneum at the ileostomy hole
2. Pass the end of the ileum under the peritoneum lateral to the caecal reflexion and burrow it extraperitoneally to the ileostomy hole. Now there is no lateral space to close

Closure

1. Close the abdominal wound in layers with appropriate drains for the procedure undertaken
2. Fashion the ileostomy spout by everting the last 2–3 cm of ileum and place several interrupted absorbable sutures between ileum and skin around its circumference
3. Place an ileostomy bag over the stoma

Postoperative management

1. Histological examination of the resected specimen
2. Control of ileostomy effluent
   a. Allow a normal diet but encourage the patient to avoid any food which upsets the stoma
   b. Usually works after each meal
   c. If too liquid, use loperamide

Complications

1. Skin excoriation
2. Retraction
3. Prolapse
4. Small bowel obstruction
   a. Adhesions
   b. Lateral space herniation

TRANSVERSE COLOSTOMY

Indications

1. Elective – defunction the descending colon and rectum
2. Emergency – as the first stage of treatment for a complete obstruction of the distal colon

Preoperative management
1. Fully informed consent, explain how the colostomy functions and (if possible) introduce the patient to the stoma therapist to explain about stoma care
2. Investigations – those relevant to the pathology
   a. Abdominal plain X-rays
   b. Sigmoidoscopy
   c. Colonoscopy } Except in perforated diverticular disease
   d. Barium enema
3. Preparation
   a. Bowel preparation if not obstructed (*see* p. 104)
   b. If obstructed, correct
      • Anaemia
      • Fluid and electrolyte balance
4. Broad spectrum and metronidazole antibiotic prophylaxis
5. Nasogastric tube
6. IVI
7. Catheter, if obstructed

Pre-incision
1. General anaesthesia with endotracheal intubation
2. Position – supine
3. Skin preparation of whole of abdomen

Incision
10 cm transverse incision in the right upper quadrant

Procedure
1. Assess the intra-peritoneal pathology by as full a laparotomy as possible via the incision
2. Locate and withdraw the transverse colon (identified by the attachment of greater omentum)
3. Locate a point on the colon proximal to the middle colic artery and detach the omentum from the colon at this point
4. Open a window at an avascular point in the mesocolon at this point and pass the plastic bridge through this hole
5. Wrap the redundant omentum around the proximal and distal limbs of the colon
6. Close the wound in layers around the prepared transverse colon with the greater omentum plugging the corners at each end. The bridge now sits outside the wound
7. Once the wound is closed around the colon, open the colon along a taenia and suture the mucosa of the colon to the skin edges with interrupted absorbable sutures
8. Secure the rod with a length of rubber tubing over each end and place a colostomy bag over the stoma

Postoperative management
1. Commence oral fluids next day and colostomy training as soon as possible
2. Remove the securing bridge after 3–4 days

Complications
1. Colostomy retraction
2. Colostomy prolapse
3. Parastomal herniation
4. Ischaemia of colostomy
5. Stomal stenosis
6. Stomal ulceration
7. Stomal obstruction
8. Faecal overflow into distal limb rendering defunctioning ineffective

CLOSURE OF TRANSVERSE COLOSTOMY

Preoperative management
1. Distal limb barium enema (to assess resolution of pathology or integrity of anastomosis)
2. Preparation of bowel including distal limb washouts
3. Nasogastric tube optional
4. IVI
5. Broad spectrum and metronidazole antibiotic prophylaxis

Pre-incision
1. Pick up the collar of parastomal skin in tissue holding forceps
2. Mobilise colostomy by incising directly through all layers to the peritoneum
3. Beware
   a. Perforating the colon, especially at the junction with the rectus sheath
   b. Perforation of an insinuated loop of small bowel
4. Excise the collar of skin and fibrous tissue from the colon by sharp dissection
5. Close the colon in two layers and return to the peritoneum

Closure in layers

Postoperative management
Commence oral fluids when flatus passed per rectum

Complications
1. Stenosis at colostomy closure (rare)
2. Leakage
   a. Faecal peritonitis
   b. Abscess
   c. Fistula (especially if closed by the extra peritoneal method)

OPERATIONS FOR COLORECTAL CARCINOMA – GENERAL PRINCIPLES

Preoperative management
1. Investigations
   a. Haemoglobin, correct anaemia if present
   b. Barium enema   } Exclude multiple primary tumours
   c. Colonoscopy with biopsy
   d. IVP to exclude ureteric involvement (large tumours of the caecum and recto-sigmoid junction)
2. Full bowel preparation
3. Broad spectrum with metronidazole antibiotic prophylaxis
4. IVI
5. Nasogastric tube
6. Catheter

Pre-incision
General anaesthesia with endotracheal intubation

Procedure
1. Full laparotomy
2. Assess the tumour operability
   a. Site and proximal obstruction
   b. Fixity (avoid undue handling)
   c. Spread
      • Locally
      • Nodes
      • Liver (intra-opreative ultrasound)
      • Peritoneum
3. Specific operation (see p. 112–121)

Postoperative management
1. Commence oral fluids at the passage of flatus per rectum/stoma
2. Continue prophylactic antibiotics parenterally for two further doses
3. Remove drain at the first passage of a solid stool

Complications
1. Early
   a. Anastomosis
      • Stricture
      • Breakdown with leakage
   b. Infection
      • Abscess
      • Peritonitis
      • Wound infection
      • Septicaemia (portal pyaemia)
   c. Haemorrhage
      • Reactionary

2. Late
   a. Obstruction
      • Adhesions
      • Anastomosis – stricture
                      local recurrence
   b. Tumour recurrence
      • Locally
      • Metastases – liver
                      peritoneum
      • New colorectal primary

RIGHT HEMICOLECTOMY

(*See* General principles, p. 111)

Pre-incision
1. Position
   Supine with 20° tilt of the table to the left – the surgeon stands
   on the left side of the patient
2. Skin preparation of all of abdomen

Incision
Right paramedian or mid-line

Procedure
1. Ligate/clamp the bowel proximally and distally to the tumour to
   reduce intraluminal spread
2. Divide the peritoneum 2 cm lateral and parallel to the colon
   from the caecum to the hepatic flexure. Mobilise the ascending
   colon medially

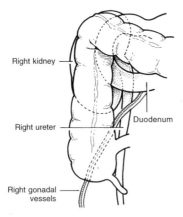

Right kidney

Right ureter

Duodenum

Right gonadal
vessels

Fig. 18 Structures to beware
during right hemicolectomy.

3. Beware (Fig. 18)
   a. Right kidney
   b. Duodenum
   c. Right ureter
   d. Right gonadal vessels
4. Elevate the bowel to expose the origin of the ileocolic artery –
   ligate and divide
   a. Right branches of middle colic vessels
   b. Right colic vessels
   c. Ileocolic vessels
   d. Vessels to last 30 cm of ileum
5. Place soft bowel clamps on ileum, 30 cm from ileocolic valve
   and at the junction of the proximal and middle third of the
   transverse colon
6. Place crushing bowel clamps 4–6 cm within the soft bowel
   clamps on the bowel to be resected
7. Divide the bowel flush with the crushing clamps and remove the
   specimen
8. Anastomose the ileum end-to-end or end-to-side with the
   transverse colon in two layers

Problems
1. Multiple secondaries
   Perform local resection of tumour to reduce the chances of
   mechanical obstruction
2. Irresectable tumour
   Ileo-transverse anastomosis

Closure in layers
(*See* General principles, p. 111)

LEFT HEMICOLECTOMY

Preoperative management
Advise the patient of the possible necessity for a defunctioning
colostomy to protect a colonic anastomosis or if a Hartmann
procedure becomes necessary (*see* General principles, p. 111 and
Hartmann procedure, p. 120)

Pre-incision
1. Position
   a. Supine with 20° tilt on the table to the right
   b. Surgeon standing on the patient's right
2. Skin preparation of all of abdomen, towel up for a left
   paramedian or mid-line incision

Incision
Left paramedian or mid-line

Procedure
1. Ligate or clamp the bowel proximally and distally to the tumour to reduce intraluminal spread as a result of operative manoeuvres
2. Incise the peritoneum 2 cm lateral to the sigmoid colon and continue upwards parallel to the descending colon including the splenic flexure
3. Divide the peritoneal reflection between the splenic flexure and the spleen (Fig. 19)
4. Beware
   a. Spleen
   b. Tail of pancreas
   c. Left kidney
   d. Left ureter
   e. Left gonadal vessels
5. Elevate the colon medially to display the inferior mesenteric vessels
6. Ligate and divide
   a. Inferior mesenteric artery, flush with the aorta (thereby resecting those lymph nodes draining the operative specimen to the pre-aortic chain of nodes en bloc with the tumour)
   b. Inferior mesenteric vein
   c. Left branch of middle colic vessels
   d. Marginal vessels at mid transverse colon
7. Place soft bowel clamps at the junction of mid-third and distal-third of transverse colon and distal sigmoid colon. Place crushing clamps 2–3 cm within these soft bowel clamps

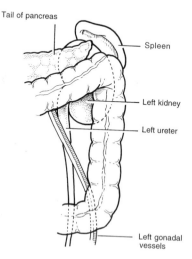

Tail of pancreas

Spleen

Left kidney

Left ureter

Left gonadal vessels

Fig. 19 Structures to beware during left hemicolectomy.

8. Divide the bowel flush with the crushing clamps and remove the specimen for histological examination
9. It may be necessary to mobilise the hepatic flexure in order to perform the colo-colonic anastomosis without tension
10. Perform an end-to-end colo-colonic anastomosis in two layers

Problems
1. Irresectable tumour – defunctioning transverse colostomy
2. Resectable tumour with multiple metastases – limited bowel resection with end-to-end anastomosis to reduce the risk of mechanical obstruction
3. Large bowel obstruction due to tumour or inadequate bowel preparation. Perform left hemicolectomy as above but protect the anastomosis with a defunctioning transverse colostomy or perform on-table colonic lavage

Closure
1. Wash out any faecal spillage with warm saline (antiseptic optional)
2. Close in layers, possibly with a non-suction drain to the anastomosis

Postoperative management
Distal limb barium enema prior to closure of defunctioning colostomy (see General principles, p. 111)

ANTERIOR RESECTION OF THE RECTUM

Indications
1. Rectal carcinoma between 5 cm from anus and the recto-sigmoid junction
2. Small resectable low primary rectal malignancy with metastases (avoids colostomy)

Preoperative management
Warn the patient of the possible need for a colostomy (defunctioning transverse or end colostomy if an abdominoperineal excision becomes necessary) (see General principles, p. 111)

Pre-incision
1. Position – lithotomy – Trendelenberg in Lloyd Davis stirrups allows access to the anus for either abdomino-perineal excision if necessary or a low rectal anastomosis using a circular EEA stapling gun
2. Skin preparation of whole of abdomen for a left paramedian incision

Incision
Long left paramedian or mid-line

Procedure
1. Pack away the small bowel and right colon, using a Golligher retractor
2. Mobilise the splenic flexure of the colon. Continue by dividing the peritoneum 2 cm lateral to the descending colon down to the sigmoid mesentery
3. Ligate and divide the inferior mesenteric vessels and their branches below the level of mid sigmoid (see Left hemicolectomy, p. 113). Continue the peritoneal incision onto both leaves of sigmoid mesentery to envelope the rectum
4. Beware left ureter as it crosses the bifurcation of the common iliac artery, deep to the apex of the sigmoid mesentery
5. Mobilise the rectum – divide
   a. The mesorectum posteriorly
   b. Lateral ligaments of the rectum
6. Beware both ureters in the pelvis as they lie adjacent to the lateral rectal ligaments. Ligate the stumps of the lateral rectal ligaments
7. The rectum is now mobilised and can be delivered into the abdomen. The tumour should be palpable
8. Place two soft bowel clamps, one across mid sigmoid colon and the other at least 3–4 cm below the tumour across the distal rectum. Place crushing clamps across the bowel 4–6 cm within the soft clamps
9. Divide the bowel flush with the crushing clamps and remove the specimen
10. Perform the anastomosis between the mobilised descending/sigmoid colon and distal rectum with either a single layer of interrupted mucosal inverting sutures or using a circular EEA stapling gun passed per anum

Closure
1. Place a non-suction drain down to the anastomosis, brought out via a separate stab incision
2. Doubt about the viability of the anastomosis, then a defunctioning transverse colostomy (see Closure of transverse colostomy, p. 110)
3. Close in layers

Postoperative management
1. Remove the pelvic drain after the passage of solid faeces through the anastomosis
2. Complications
   a. Early – acute retention of urine
   b. Late – anastomotic stricture – treat by rectal dilatation (see General principles, p. 111)

ABDOMINO-PERINEAL EXCISION OF THE RECTUM

Indications
1. Carcinoma of the rectum within 6 cm of the anus
2. Carcinoma of the anus (*see* General principles, p. 111)

Preoperative management
Fully informed consent about the nature of the colostomy, introduce the patient to the stoma therapist and mark the site of the colostomy midway between the anterior superior iliac spine and the umbilicus in the standing, sitting and lying position, the final position being a compromise of the three, avoiding skin creases

Pre-incision
1. Position – lithotomy – Trendelenberg with Lloyd Davis stirrups. The shoulders and sacrum should be well supported
2. Skin preparation of all of abdomen and perineum. Towel up each leg separately and cover the genitals, leaving the perineum and abdomen exposed
3. Position of operators
   a. Abdominal operator on the left, assistant on the right
   b. Perineal operating sitting, facing the perineum
4. Perineal operator
   Purse-string with a stout silk suture around the anus and tie off to reduce faecal spillage

Incision
Commence with a low left paramedian or mid-line incision

Abdominal operator procedure
1. Full laparotomy, with special regard to the tumour (*see* General principles, p. 111). If the tumour is resectable then allow the perineal operator to commence
2. Pack away the small bowel towards the right hypochondrium and retract the wound edges with a self retaining retractor (e.g. Golligher's)
3. Mobilise the sigmoid colon by dividing the peritoneum 1–2 cm lateral to it, down as far as the rectum
4. Beware the left ureter as it crosses the bifurcation of the common iliac artery, deep to the apex of the sigmoid mesentery
5. Divide the right leaf of the pelvic mesocolon as it descends around the upper third of the rectum
6. Beware the adjacent right ureter
7. Ligate and divide the inferior mesenteric vessels
8. Select the level of transection on the descending colon and clean the appendices epiploicae off the bowel. Place a soft bowel clamp across the bowel and a crushing clamp 2 cm distal to this

9. Divide the bowel flush with the crushing clamp
10. Mobilise the rectum by dividing the posterior mesorectum
11. Beware the presacral plexus
12. Ligate and divide the lateral ligaments of the rectum containing the middle rectal vessels
13. Beware the ureters lying laterally
14. In the male
    a. Divide the fascia of Denonvilliers anteriorly
    b. Beware the seminal vesicles anteriorly
15. In the female incise the posterior wall of the vagina jointly with the perineal operator

Perineal operator procedure
1. Incision
   Elliptical commencing at the coccyx and passing 2 cm lateral to the anal verge and finishing:
   a. Male – at the perineal body
   b. Female – at the posterior wall of the vagina
2. Place a self retaining retractor within the wound
3. Deepen the incision
   a. Posteriorly to the mesorectum to meet the abdominal operator through Waldeyer's fascia
   b. Hook the index finger of the left hand around the posterior edge of the levator ani muscles and divide the muscles with scissors immediately lateral to the index finger, clamping and ligating bleeding points
4. Retracting on the anus with a strong pair of tissue holding forceps, commence the anterior dissection
   a. Male – palpate the urethral catheter lying in the bulbar urethra, carefully dissect upwards in the plane of the fascia of Denonvilliers using scissors
   b. Female – excise the posterior wall of the vagina to the posterior fornix
5. The rectum is now completely free and is delivered to the perineal operator with the upper end clamped off by the crushing clamp

Abdominal operator closure
1. Create a 3 cm diameter all layers circular incision at the predetermined site for the colostomy. Deliver the mobilised free end of the descending colon through this incision
2. No intra-abdominal drains
3. Close the pelvic peritoneum over the defect, if this is not possible then mobilise the greater omentum off the transverse colon on a pedicle based on the left gastro-epiploic artery, and deliver it to the pelvis through a window in the transverse mesocolon and pack the pelvis
4. Close the abdominal wound in layers

5. Fashion the end colostomy using 8–10 interrupted absorbable mucocutaneous sutures
6. Place a colostomy bag over the stoma

Perineal operator closure
1. Absolute haemostasis is very important
2. Place a suction drain into the pelvic defect
3. Close the levator ani muscles
4. Close the perineal skin

Problems
Continuing bleeding
1. Moderate bleeding – pack the defect with a polythene sheet held in place by a long gauze roll pack which can be gradually shortened as the wound is allowed to granulate
2. Severe bleeding – this is usually a consequence of a tear in a large median sacral vein. Consider ligation of the internal iliac vessels by the abdominal operator or radiological embolisation. Alternatively, consider tamponade of the vein using drawing pins pushed through the torn vein, embedded in the sacrum

Postoperative management
1. Remove the perineal drain when drainage is minimal
2. Remove the catheter after 3–4 days. Haematuria after this procedure is very common in males as a result of blunt trauma to the bladder
3. Commence colostomy training as soon as possible with continuing psychological support

Complications
1. Early
   a. Infection
      • Wound infection
      • Pelvic abscess
   b. Colostomy (*see* Transverse colostomy, p. 108)
   c. Genito-urinary
      • Haematuria
      • Retention, especially in males 10% is permanent due to either prostatism or neurological damage during the procedure
      • Impotence
      • Fistula – uretero-perineal
               – urethra-perineal
2. Late
   a. Tumour recurrence (*see* General principles, p. 111)
   b. Pelvic recurrence may present as sciatica

HARTMANN'S OPERATION

Indications
1. Obstructing carcinoma at the recto-sigmoid junction, especially in the elderly
2. Perforation of a sigmoid diverticulum with gross inflammatory change of the adjacent colon
3. First stage of surgery for sigmoid volvulus

Preoperative management
1. This operation is performed in the emergency situation on unprepared bowel so warn the patient of the subsequent colostomy
2. Resuscitate
   a. Correct
      • Electrolytes
      • Anaemia
   b. Commence antibiotics (broad spectrum and metronidazole)
3. IVI
   a. Peripheral for fluid replacement
   b. Central to monitor fluid replacement
4. Nasogastric tube
   Aspirate gastric contents, as these patients are at grave risk from aspiration
5. Catheterise
   To empty the bladder and subsequently monitor urine output

Pre-incision
1. General anaesthetic with endotracheal intubation
2. Position – supine with a slight Trendelenberg tilt
3. Skin preparation of all abdomen and towel up for a left paramedian incision

Incision
Lower left paramedian

Procedure
1. Assess the problem
   a. Obstructing carcinoma – assess the degree of obstruction and the tumour (see General principles, p. 111)
   b. Perforated diverticular disease
      • Mop out all faecal contamination and perform a full peritoneal toilet
      • Sample for microbiological examination
   c. Sigmoid volvulus – reduce the volvulus
2. Mobilise the sigmoid colon (fibrous adhesions may arise around either a tumour or diverticular disease)
3. Divide and ligate the branches of the inferior mesenteric vessels to the sigmoid colon

4. Divide the peritoneal reflection from the sigmoid mesentery as it descends around the upper third of the rectum and mobilise the upper third of the rectum
5. Beware damage to the left ureter
6. Place a soft bowel clamp across the lower descending colon and a second soft bowel clamp across the upper third of the rectum. Place crushing clamps 2 cm within these on the bowel to be resected
7. Divide the sigmoid colon flush with the crushing clamps and remove the specimen
8. Close the rectal stump in two layers

Closure
1. If there has been gross pelvic contamination then leave a drain to the pelvis after completion of the peritoneal lavage
2. Bring the distal descending colon out through a 3 cm diameter circular incision lying midway between the anterior superior iliac spine and the umbilicus. Keep the soft bowel clamp in place until the abdomen is closed
3. Close in layers
4. Create the colostomy with 8–10 interrupted circumferential absorbable sutures
5. Place a colostomy bag over the stoma

Postoperative management
1. Commence oral fluid at the return of bowel sounds and solid food after the colostomy has passed faeces
2. Remove the pelvic drain when drainage is minimal and the track has started to granulate (approximately 5 days)
3. Investigations
   a. Histological examination of the specimen
   b. Microbiology results
4. Subsequent reconnection of the descending colon to the rectal stump should be undertaken once the patient's condition has improved sufficiently to tolerate the procedure. The use of circular (EEA) stapling gun for this has been described.

Complications
1. Those of colostomy (*see* Transverse colostomy, p. 108)
2. Infection
   a. Pelvic abscess
   b. Wound infection
   c. Septicaemia

IVALON SPONGE REPAIR FOR COMPLETE RECTAL PROLAPSE

Indications
Complete rectal prolapse (intussusception) in the elderly with no other pathological cause

Preoperative management
1. Investigations
   a. Barium enema/colonoscopy to exclude pathological cause for prolapse, especially intussusception of the rectum with a polyp/tumour (in this situation defaecating proctography and anorectal manometry may also be of assistance)
   b. Sigmoidoscopy
   c. Galvanic studies of the perineal musculature
   d. Urodynamic studies to assess bladder emptying
2. Full bowel preparation (see Principles of bowel preparation, p. 104)
3. Broad spectrum with metronidazole antibiotic prophylaxis
4. IVI
5. Catheterise the bladder

Pre-incision
1. General anaesthetic with endotracheal intubation
2. Position – supine
3. Skin preparation of all of abdomen for a left paramedian incision

Incision
Left paramedian or mid-line

Procedure
1. Full laparotomy and pack the small bowel into the right hypochondrium
2. Incise the peritoneum on both sides of the sigmoid mesocolon and continue down around the upper third of the rectum to mobilise the rectum and rectosigmoid colon
3. Divide the mesorectum posteriorly for the whole length of the rectum
4. Beware the presacral plexus
5. Ligate and divide the lateral rectal ligaments containing the middle rectal vessels
6. Beware the ureters laterally
7. Mobilise the peritoneum anteriorly in the Pouch of Douglas as this forms the hernial sac which allows the prolapse to occur. Expose the vaginal vault musculature, the rectum is now fully mobilised
8. Cut the piece of Ivalon sponge to conform with the normal anatomy and envelop the rectum (usually about 20 × 10 cm)
9. Suture the tail of the sponge to the presacral fascia at the level of the sacrococcygeal junction with a nylon suture
10. Allow the rectum to fall back into the sacrococcygeal curve and wrap the Ivalon around the rectum, suturing its four free corners to the anterior rectal muscle with single nylon sutures

11. Suture the uppermost part of the mesorectum to the fascia overlying the lumbosacral disc with a nylon suture
12. Extraperitonealise the rectum by closing the pelvic peritoneum over it

Closure
1. No drains
2. Close in layers

Postoperative management
1. Commence oral fluids at the return of bowel sounds and solids after the passage of faeces
2. Long-term use of bulk laxatives or hydrophilic laxative may be necessary
3. Perform regular rectal examinations in the postoperative period to prevent faecal impaction

Complications
1. Early
   a. Infection
      • Around the prosthesis as a result of foreign material implantation
      • Wound infection (although the bowel is not opened)
   b. DVT – pelvic surgery in an elderly patient (*see* Principles of prevention, p. 7)
   c. Faecal impaction
2. Late
   a. Recurrent prolapse – <10%
   b. Anal incontinence due to anal sphincter weakness may need a post-anal repair

PRINCIPLES OF HAEMORRHOID SURGERY

Management
1. Exclude predisposing anorectal pathology, especially carcinoma of the rectum
2. Proctoscopy to examine the anal canal and haemorrhoids
3. Sigmoidoscopy to examine the rectum
4. Haemoglobin, as blood loss can be significant

FIRST DEGREE

No prolapse, but bleeding and discharge causes pruritic ani. Treat by submucosal injection of 5 ml of 5% phenol in almond oil immediately above the haemorrhoid and therefore above the dentate line (the limit of somatic sensation)

SECOND DEGREE

Prolapse but withdraw spontaneously
Treat by banding with tight rubber bands (Barron)
Withdraw the haemorrhoid via the proctoscope with Barron's
grasping forceps which have been passed through the band
applicator
Apply the band by releasing the band applicator over the base of
the haemorrhoid, ensuring that this will be constricted above the
dentate line

THIRD DEGREE – HAEMORRHOIDECTOMY

Preoperative management

Preparation – two disposable enemata, one the day before and one
immediately prior to surgery

Pre-incision

1. General anaesthetic with endotracheal intubation
2. Position – lithotomy
3. Skin preparation of perineum and anal canal
4. Surgeon sitting facing the perineum
5. Pick up the haemorrhoid and inject a solution of 1:100 000
   adrenaline submucosally beneath the haemorrhoid, raising it
   from the internal sphincter muscle in a relatively bloodless field

Procedure

1. Insert Parkes anal speculum to display the haemorrhoid to be
   operated upon
2. Grasp the haemorrhoid with a haemostatic forcep and retract
   towards the surgeon
3. Incise the skin at the base of the haemorrhoid with scissors as a
   V-shaped incision
4. Extend this incision into the mucosa either side of the
   haemorrhoid raising it off the muscles of the internal sphincter
5. Transfix and ligate the pedicle of the haemorrhoid with a silk
   suture leaving a long length of suture material attached. Excise
   the haemorrhoid 0.5 cm distal to the ligature
6. Repeat the procedure with the other haemorrhoids
7. Leave a mucocutaneous bridge between each haemorrhoid to
   reduce any subsequent anal stricture
8. At the end place a small paraffin soaked pack to reduce bleeding
   within the anal canal, supported by a T-shaped bandage

Postoperative management

1. Encourage bowel action with adequate analgesia and bulk
   laxative
2. Digital rectal examination at the fifth postoperative day to
   exclude anal stenosis (if suspected, then commence the daily
   use of an anal dilator)

Complications
1. Early
   a. Haemorrhage – reactionary
   b. Acute retention of urine
   c. Constipation with pain resulting in faecal impaction
2. Late
   a. Anal stenosis
   b. Fissure
   c. Skin tags
   d. Recurrent haemorrhoids
   e. Incontinence with sphincter damage

TREATMENT OF ANAL FISSURE

Chronic anal fissures either lie posteriorly (90% in men, 60% in women) or anteriorly (10% in men, 40% in women) they must be differentiated from
1. Carcinoma of the anus
2. Anal chancre
3. TB
4. Herpes
A careful search must be made for evidence of Crohn's disease, and less commonly, ulcerative colitis

MANUAL DILATATION OF THE ANUS (LORD PROCEDURE)

Contraindications (and therefore not recommended by the author)
1. Patulous anus with mucosal prolapse
2. Fibrous anal stricture
3. Caution in the elderly since this may produce a complete rectal prolapse

Preoperative management
Rectal washout prior to surgery

Preprocedure
(In the left lateral position)
(i) General anaesthetic with an endotracheal tube as this procedure may induce laryngospasm
(ii) Perform an examination under anaesthesia with a full sigmoidoscopy to exclude other pathology

Procedure
(i)   Proceeding gently, insert the index and third fingers of each hand and dilate the internal sphincter laterally, relaxing and breaking down the spasm and fibrosis induced by the fissure
(ii) Maintain for 3–4 minutes
(iii) At the end place a small anal pack which is withdrawn once the patient is awake

Postoperative management
(i) Commence on a bulk laxative the next day and continue using a daily anal dilator for 1 month
(ii) Complications
   a. Tearing (splitting of the anal canal)
   b. Mucosal prolapse
   c. Incontinence

LATERAL SPHINCTEROTOMY

Preoperative management
Rectal washout prior to surgery

Pre-procedure
1. Either general or local anaesthetic (1% Xylocaine with 1 in 200 000 adrenaline) 5 ml into the base of the fissure and 5 ml at 3 o'clock on the anal verge
2. Left lateral position
3. Sigmoidoscopy to exclude co-existing pathology

Procedure
1. Insert the left index finger into the anal canal
2. Insert the blade of the sphincterotomy knife through the skin at the anal margin and pass it up in the subcutaneous tissue with the blade flat and parallel to the mucosa for 2–3 cm
3. Rotate the cutting blade of the knife through 90° away from the lumen and divide the lower fibres of the internal sphincter. There will be a palpable 'give' when this is achieved
4. Remove the knife and press to prevent haematoma formation

Postoperatively
Commence on a bulk laxative to soften the stool

Complications
1. Incontinence if the external sphincter is also inadvertently divided
2. Perianal haematoma
3. Recurrent fissure

SURGERY FOR FISTULA IN ANO

PATHOLOGICAL PRINCIPLES

Goodsall's rule
1. All fistulae anterior to a coronal plane through the centre of the anus track radially to the recto-anal canal
2. All fistulae posterior to this plane track circumferentially to enter the anorectal canal in the midline posteriorly

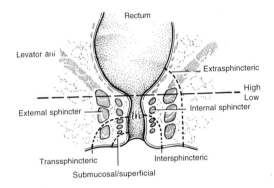

Fig. 20 Parkes' classification of low and high fistulae in ano.

Parkes' classification (Fig. 20)

1. Low (95%)
   a. Submucosal/superficial
   b. Intersphincteric
   c. Transsphincteric
2. High (5%)
   a. Suprasphincteric
   b. Extrasphincteric

Simple versus complicated

1. Simple
   Direct track, not involving any sphincter, to the mucosa, although no internal opening is necessarily present
2. Complicated
   Multiple perianal tracks or a high fistula

Exclude co-existent or causative pathology

1. Crohn's disease
2. Carcinoma
3. TB

SIMPLE LOW FISTULAE

Preoperative management

Rectal washout prior to surgery

Procedure

1. General anaesthetic
2. Position – lithotomy
3. Pass a probe from the fistula opening towards the anus; if there is no inner opening then push the probe through into the anal lumen

4. Excise the fistula, leaving a wide gap between the skin/mucosa on each side to prevent 'bridging' resulting in a recurrent fistula
5. Send the specimen for histological examination
6. Dress and support this with a T-bandage

Postoperative management
1. Daily bulk laxative and simple analgesia
2. Histological examination of the specimen

COMPLICATED/HIGH FISTULA
1. Exclude underlying pathology (carcinoma and Crohn's disease)
2. Consider defunctioning the anus with a transverse colostomy (*see* p. 108) prior to definitive surgery
3. Treatment is best undertaken in specialist centres and involves excision of the fistula track, defining the sphincter layers in the process and reconstruction of these layers as a primary or secondary procedure
4. Alternatively, pass an absorbable suture (silk/nylon) through the length of the fistula and then tie the two ends together outside the anus. Gradually pull this through the layers encouraging fibrosis along its track and allowing drainage along the length of the suture

Complications
1. Recurrent fistulae and abscesses
2. Faecal incontinence if a high fistula is treated inappropriately and the external sphincter is divided

PILONIDAL SINUS

Preoperative management
1. Carefully examine the natal cleft and locate all the openings both within the cleft and also laterally
2. Beware confusion with fistula in ano
Antibiotic prophylaxis is unnecessary

Pre-incision
1. Either general or local (Xylocaine with adrenaline) anaesthetic
2. Position – lateral or prone with buttocks abducted
3. Skin preparation of natal cleft to anus and both buttocks

Procedure
1. Meticulously shave the region around the sinuses
2. Gently probe and delineate all tracks
3. Excise the midline pits in an elliptical incision
4. Excise the lateral sinuses with a small circumference of surrounding skin
5. Curette out the sinus tracks

Closure
Either
1. Regular dry dressings or silastic foam dressing and allow to granulate
   or
2. Primary closure

Postoperative management
Continue regular weekly shaving area adjacent to and including the sinus wound

PILONIDAL ABSCESS

1. Excise the roof as for pilonidal sinus
2. Pus specimen for microbiological analysis
3. Allow to granulate, avoid primary closure

SURGERY FOR PERIANAL AND ISCHIORECTAL ABSCESS

Pathological principles
Abscesses in this region follow the same anatomical principles as fistulae (Fig. 21). They can be classified as
 • Perianal
 • Submucosal
 • Intersphincteric
 • Ischiorectal
 • Pelvic (pararectal)
These abscesses may be associated with a history of perianal sepsis and fistula

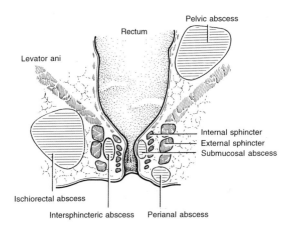

Fig. 21 Anatomy of perianal and ischiorectal abscesses.

Procedure

1. General anaesthetic (although superficial perianal abscesses can be drained successfully under local anaesthetic)
2. Lithotomy position
3. Perform a proctoscopy and sigmoidoscopy to exclude an internal fistula opening
4. Make a cruciform incision over the place where the abscess is pointing
5. Release the pus, sending a specimen for culture and sensitivity
6. Gently break down any internal loculi
7. Wash out and gently pack with calcium alginate. May ultimately take a silastic dressing if some distance from the anal verge

Pelvic abscesses may be drained via the rectum, by passing a finger through the rectal wall at the place where the abscess is pointing

Urology

URETHRAL CATHETERISATION

Objective
1. Diagnostic, therefore not self-retaining (short term, temporary or long term silastic intermittent self catheterisation)
2. Therapeutic
   a. Urethral – smallest self retaining
   b. Suprapubic
3. Indications for a large bore catheter
   a. Clots
   b. Infected urine

Preparation
1. Position – supine
2. Prepare the genitals with antiseptic, retracting the foreskin fully
3. Strict asepsis is essential
4. Local anaesthetic to urethra
5. Select catheter size

Procedure
1. Pass the appropriate catheter gently, without force
2. Once in position
   a. Attach to a closed collecting system
   b. Inflate self-retaining balloon

Complications
1. Unable to pass catheter – use either
   a. Narrower catheter
   b. Beaked Coude catheter
   c. Catheter introducer
   d. Suprapubic catheter
   e. *Or seek assistance*
2. Significant haematuria
   Consider replacing with a larger 3-way irrigating catheter

URETHRAL DILATATION

Preoperative management
1. Investigations
   a. MSU for MC&S
   b. Urethrogram
2. Correct pre-existing urinary tract infection
3. Empty the bladder immediately prior to the procedure
4. Antibiotic cover is essential if there has been a recent urinary tract infection
5. Use either general or local (Xylocaine gel) anaesthetic

Procedure
1. Position – supine
2. Strict asepsis essential
3. Meatal stricture
   a. Use either Hegar's dilator or female urethral dilator
   b. Start with the largest dilator which is passable with no resistance
   c. *Never* force the dilator
   d. Cease as soon as bleeding commences
4. Urethral stricture
   Use either Clutton's or Liston's bougies
5. Notation on bougie
   <u>Circumference at tip in mm (French gauge)</u>
   Circumference of shaft in mm (French gauge)
6. Always pass without force with the beak pointing dorsally on the penis
7. Beware false passages
8. Continue, using next larger size until the bougie is gripped; never force beyond this point
9. Cease as soon as bleeding commences

Complications
Failure to pass bougie
1. Try a smaller size (<14F use gum elastic bougie)
2. If this fails, use filiforms (*faggoti* method with a follower)
3. Refer to a urologist for urethroplasty

Postoperative management
MSU after procedure

Complications
1. False passage
2. Infection
   a. Ascending urinary tract infection
   b. Septicaemia
3. Stricture
   a. Recurrent
   b. Iatrogenic due to traumatic dilatation

CYSTOSCOPY, LITHOLOPAXY AND RETROGRADE URETEROGRAPHY

Preoperative management
1. Investigation
   a. MSU – correct UTI if present
   b. IVP
2. Antibiotic cover if urine recently infected

Pre-procedure
1. Spinal, epidural or general anaesthetic (endotracheal tube if endoscopic resection anticipated)
2. Position – lithotomy
3. Skin preparation of all of external genitalia, retracting foreskin with a drape over the suprapubic area to allow palpation of the bladder

CYSTOSCOPY

Procedure
1. Urethroscopy using a 30° telescope in the irrigating sheath down the urethra with no force
2. Remove the obturator, empty the bladder, measuring the urine volume and collecting a specimen for microbiological examination
3. Irrigate the bladder with isotonic saline solution, evacuate any clots or debris
4. Pass the 70° telescope with light source attached and visualise the distending bladder
5. Examine the distended bladder, noting the air bubble, ureteric orifices, trigone and prostatic impression (Marion's sign)
6. Remove the telescope, empty the bladder and replace the obturator prior to removal of the sheath
7. Finish the procedure with a bimanual examination of the pelvis

LITHOLOPAXY

Contraindications
1. Children <10 years old
2. Infected urine
3. Urethral stricture
4. Bladder pathology
   a. Diverticulum
   b. Carcinoma
   c. Tuberculosis
   d. Bilharzia

Needs
1. Antibiotic cover
2. General anaesthetic with endotracheal intubation

Procedure
1. Pass the lithotrite, beak anteriorly into the bladder, insert a 30° telescope and fill the bladder with irrigating fluid
2. Visualise the stone and grasp it in the blades of the lithotrite
3. Crush the stone into small fragments, withdraw the lithotrite, insert an irrigating sheath and irrigate the stone fragments for biochemical analysis

RETROGRADE URETEROGRAPHY

Indications
1. Delineation of the lower limit of a complete ureteric obstruction
2. Pyelography in a poorly functioning kidney

Procedure
1. Pass the catheterising cystoscope and visualise the ureteric orifices and trigone
2. Difficulty may arise in a very trabeculated bladder
3. Gently pass a straight ureteric catheter (size 3F) up the ureter as far as the level to be visualised
4. Withdraw the stillette and cystoscope, collect urine for cytological examination in suspected malignancy
5. Pyelography/ureterography by injection of Hypaque either in theatre using an image intensifier or transferring the patient to the X-ray department
6. Remove ureteric catheter immediately after the procedure to reduce the risk of ascending infection

Postoperative management
1. MSU
2. Litholopaxy – 3-way irrigating catheter

Complications
1. Infection
   a. Urinary tract
   b. Septicaemia
2. Bladder perforation
   a. Intraperitoneal – laparotomy
   b. Extraperitoneal
      • Minor – catheterise
      • Major – laparotomy
3. Urethral stricture
4. Ureteric perforation

PRINCIPLES OF TRANSURETHRAL RESECTION OF PROSTATE (TURP)

Preoperative management

1. Investigations
   a. MSU – treat existing urinary tract infection
   b. IVP/ultrasound to assess residual urine volume and upper track dilatation
   c. Tartrate labile acid phosphatase
   d. Prostate specific antigen (PSA)
   e. Renal function
   f. Urodynamic studies to show flow rate
2. IVI
3. Antibiotic prophylaxis for Gram-negative organisms
4. Explain the consequences of subsequent retrograde ejaculation

Pre-procedure

1. Either general or epidural anaesthetic
2. Position – lithotomy
3. Prepare as for cystoscopy (*see* p.133)

Procedure

1. Select a resectoscope sheath which will pass down the urethra without force
2. Problem – small meatus, perform meatotomy
3. Perform a cystoscopy and urethroscopy (*see* p.133) to exclude co-existent bladder pathology
4. Pass the resectoscope
5. Irrigate with isotonic glycine (systemic entry of irrigation fluid will occur at the prostatic bed, isotonic solutions prevent red cell osmotic lysis, glycine equilibrates throughout the total body water and reduces the risk of cardiac overload)
6. Insert the resectoscope with a 30° telescope
7. Commence resection
   a. First – circumferential resection of the bladder neck
   b. Then resect the lateral lobes distally as far as the verumontanum
   c. Never resect beyond the pink transverse fibres of the prostatic capsule or resect distal to the verumontanum
8. Coagulate all bleeding vessels as they arise
9. Using the irrigating resectoscope at intervals wash out the prostatic chipping from the bladder and send for histological examination
10. At the end of the procedure, insert a three-way irrigation catheter (22–24F) into the bladder and irrigate with glycine solution until the haematuria has subsided

Complications
1. Early
   a. Infection
      - Urine
      - Septicaemia
   b. Bleeding
      - Reactionary
      - Secondary – urinary infection
                         carcinoma of the prostate
2. Late
   a. Recurrence of 'prostatism'
      - Inadequate resection
      - Urethral stricture
      - Bladder neck stenosis
   b. Recurrent carcinoma
   c. Metastatic carcinoma
   d. Impotence
   e. Incontinence
   f. Retrograde ejaculation

RETROPUBIC PROSTATECTOMY

Preoperative management
1. Investigations as for TURP (*see* p.135)
2. IVI
3. Antibiotic prophylaxis to Gram-negative bacteria

Pre-incision
1. General anaesthetic with endotracheal intubation
2. Position
   a. Initially lithotomy, perform cystoscopy to exclude co-existent bladder pathology
   b. Then supine with Trendelenberg tilt of 5° – surgeon standing on the left side
3. Skin preparation for a low abdominal incision with penis prepared and accessible

Incision
Transverse suprapubic (Pfannenstiel)

Procedure
1. Divide the linea alba and insert Millin's retractor to expose the cave of Retzius, depress the bladder with the third blade
2. Place two small swabs, one each side in the lateral limits of the retropubic space
3. Stay sutures to the prostatic capsule above and below the line of incision

4. Incise the prostate capsule transversely 1–2 cm below the vesico-prostatic junction. Control capsular bleeding
5. Divide the upper prostatic urethra with scissors and digitally enucleate the prostatic adenoma
6. Remove the adenoma after division of the lower prostatic urethra
7. Using Millin's bladder neck spreader visualise and excise the posterior overhanging bladder neck with any residual middle prostatic lobe

Closure
1. Pass an irrigating 3-way catheter per urethra into the bladder and inflate the balloon
2. Close the anterior prostatic capsule with absorbable sutures
3. Suction drain to the retropubic space
4. Close in layers
5. During the closure irrigate the bladder with citrate solution to evacuate clots

Postoperative management
As for TURP (*see* p. 135) except – remove retropubic drain after urine has been successfully passed following removal of the catheter

Complications
As for TURP (*see* p. 135) – in addition
Early
    a. DVT (pelvic surgery in the elderly)
    b. Osteitis pubis

APPROACH TO THE KIDNEY

ANTERIOR APPROACH

Position – supine

Incision
Paramedian/Kocher's subcostal on the appropriate side
Full laparotomy

Procedure
1. Divide peritoneal reflection lateral to colon and mobilise the colonic flexure
2. Beware
    a. On right
      • Hepatic flexure
      • Duodenum
      • Gonadal vessels

b. On left
   • Splenic flexure
   • Spleen
   • Tail of pancreas
   • Gonadal vessels
3. Mobilise the colon medially to display the perinephric fascia which is opened to display the kidney
4. Structures at the hilum
   a. Renal vein is most anterior
   b. Renal artery
   c. Ureter is deep to the artery
   Postoperatively ileus common

POSTERIOR APPROACH

Position lateral, with a renal bridge on the operating table under the opposite loin

Incision
1. Either supracostal or subcostal, following the line of the 12th rib; commencing 6 cm lateral to the mid-line and finishing in the posterior axillary line
2. Deepen by dividing
   a. Latissimus dorsi
   b. External oblique
   c. Internal oblique/quadratus lumborum in the line of the incision to display the perinephric fascia
   d. Identify the ureter
3. Open the perinephric fascia to display the kidney
4. Structures at the hilum
   a. Ureter is most posterior
   b. Renal artery
   c. Renal vein deep to the artery
5. Beware pneumothorax
6. Ileus common with retroperitoneal trauma

NEPHRECTOMY

Indications
1. Malignant tumour arising within the kidney
2. Chronic pyelonephritis complicated by hypertension, recurrent infection
3. Transitional cell carcinoma of the ureter treated by nephro-ureterectomy

Preoperative management
1. Examine and mark the side

2. Investigations
   a. MSU and treat concurrent urinary tract infection
   b. IVP/ultrasound/CT
      • Delineate pathology
      • Confirm the presence of opposite kidney
   c. Adenocarcinoma
      • Arteriography ± embolisation
      • Consider cavagram to exclude venous extension
   d. Transitional cell carcinoma – cystoscopy to exclude co-existing bladder tumours
   e. Urine cytology
3. Antibiotic prophylaxis to Gram-negative bacteria
4. IVI
5. Catheterise

Pre-incision
General anaesthetic with endotracheal intubation

Procedure
1. Use anterior approach (see p. 137) but do not open perinephric fascia when operating for cancer
2. Clamp the renal artery
3. Ligate and divide in continuity
   a. Renal vein (oversew the short right renal vein)
   b. Renal artery
4. Adenocarcinoma of the kidney/chronic pyelonephritis – ligate and divide ureter at an accessible point. Remove kidney for histological examination
5. Transitional cell carcinoma of the renal pelvis – needs a complete ureterectomy with excision of the vesico-ureteric junction and formal closure of the bladder

Closure
1. Large suction drain to the renal bed
2. Close in layers

Postoperative management
Investigation
1. MSU
2. Histological examination of specimen
3. Transitional cell carcinoma – needs long-term cystoscopic follow-up

Complications
1. Early
   a. Infection
      • Urine
      • Wound
      • Septicaemia

  b. Haemorrhage – reactionary at renal pedicle
  c. Ileus
  d. DVT
2. Late
  Tumour recurrence, new primary with transitional cell carcinoma

PYELOLITHOTOMY/URETEROLITHOTOMY

Preoperative management
1. Examine and mark the side
2. Investigations
   a. MSU, treat pre-existing urinary tract infection
   b. IVP
   c. Those for renal calculi (24 h urine for calcium, oxalate, urate, xanthine, cysteine analysis)
   d. Renal function (electrolytes, clearance studies)
   e. *Plain abdominal X-ray en route to the operating theatre to see if the stone has moved*
3. Broad spectrum antibiotic prophylaxis
4. IVI

Pre-incision
1. General anaesthetic with endotracheal intubation
2. Position – lateral for pyelolithotomy, supine for ureterolithotomy

PYELOLITHOTOMY

(Stone in pelvis/upper ureter)

Incision
Posterior approach (*see* p. 138)

Procedure
1. Assess and gently mobilise the kidney (beware perinephric inflammation and fibrosis)
2. Controlling the stone with the left hand retract the renal sinus with a Gilvernet retractor
3. Incise the renal pelvis over the stone in its long axis and remove the stone with Desjardins forceps. Wash out pelvis
4. On table pyelogram
5. Close the renal pelvis with interrupted absorbable sutures
6. Send the stone for biochemical analysis

Closure
1. Drains
   a. One to the renal pelvis
   b. One to the wound
2. Close in layers

URETEROLITHOTOMY
(Stones in middle third of ureter)

Incision
1. Extended grid iron in iliac fossa
2. Do not open peritoneum

Procedure
1. Sweep the peritoneum medially and locate the ureter
2. Place slings around the ureter above and below the stone
3. Gently milk the stone proximally as there may be ulceration/fibrosis of the ureter where it has impacted
4. Incise onto the stone and remove it for biochemical analysis
5. Pass a ureteric catheter distally to exclude distal obstruction
6. Close the ureter with absorbable suture

Closure
1. Drain the retroperitoneal space
2. Close in layers

Postoperative management
1. Remove the drain when drainage is minimal
2. Investigations
   a. Biochemical analysis of stones
   b. MSU

Complications
1. Early
   a. Infection
   • Urine
   • Septicaemia
   b. Stone fragmented during removal
   • Small (<1 cm) fragments should pass spontaneously
   • Larger irretrievable fragments, refer to specialist centre
   c. Hydronephrosis
   • Ureteric oedema
   • Residual calculous obstruction
2. Late
   a. Recurrent calculi
   b. Hydronephrosis
   • Ureteric stricture
   • Recurrent calculi

PRINCIPLES OF PYELOPLASTY

Indications
Idiopathic pelvic ureteric junction (PUJ) obstruction

Preoperative management
1. Examine and mark the side
2. Investigations
   a. MSU
   b. IVP
   c. Isotope renogram to assess the effect of the obstruction on renal function
3. Antibiotic prophylaxis for Gram-negative bacteria
4. IVI

Procedure
1. General anaesthetic with endotracheal intubation
2. Use posterior approach to the kidney (*see* p. 138)
3. Needs a full exposure of the kidney and pelvis
4. Type of pyeloplasty depends on the size of the renal pelvis
5. Large baggy pelvis – Anderson – Hynes pyeloplasty (Fig. 22)
   a. Divide the ureter just below the PUJ
   b. Excise the baggy redundant renal pelvis 1–2 cm from and parallel to the renal sinus
   c. Close the upper two-thirds of the renal pelvis with an absorbable continuous suture
   d. Incise the opened end of the upper ureter longitudinally on its lateral side to match the size of the opening in the lower third of the renal pelvis
   e. Pass a nephrostomy tube through the anastomosis
   f. Anastomose the upper ureter to the lower third of the renal pelvis
6. Moderate pelvis – Culp pyeloplasty (Fig. 23)
   a. Make a 6 cm longitudinal incision equidistant either side of the PUJ
   b. At the top of this incision curve it round medially and then continue it back down to the PUJ, 1 cm medial and parallel to the first incision to fashion a pedicled flap based on the PUJ

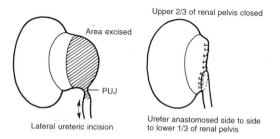

Fig. 22 Anderson–Hynes pyeloplasty.

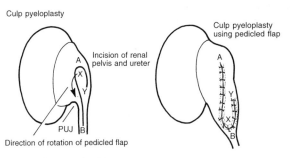

Culp pyeloplasty

Incision of renal pelvis and ureter

Culp pyeloplasty using pedicled flap

PUJ

Direction of rotation of pedicled flap

Fig. 23 Culp pyeloplasty.

   c. Rotate this flap through 180° to point inferiorly and suture onto the lower part of the incision below the PUJ with continuous absorbable sutures

   d. Close the defect in the PUJ from where the flap originated with continuous absorbable sutures

7. Small pelvis – Foley pyeloplasty
   a. Make a Y-shaped incision with the lower vertical arm commencing just above the PUJ and extending for 2 cm beyond it down the ureter
   b. Convert it to a V-shaped incision (Y-V plasty) and close with a continuous absorbable suture

Closure
1. Splint the pyeloplasty with a Malecot catheter brought out as a nephrostomy
2. Suction drain to the renal bed
3. Close in layers, draining the wound

Postoperative management
1. Remove the drain when dry
2. Remove the nephrostomy tube 10 days postoperatively
3. Investigate
   a. MSU
   b. IVP to assess pyeloplasty

Complications
1. Infection
   a. Urine
   b. Wound
   c. Septicaemia
2. Pyeloplasty leakage
   a. Usually close spontaneously
3. Recurrent obstruction

a. Usually oedema
b. Rarely, recurrent PUJ obstruction or fibrosis

PRINCIPLES OF RENAL TRANSPLANTATION

Donors – 20% live related

1. From immediate family
   a. Non-diabetic
   b. Healthy and normotensive
   c. Two normal kidneys
      • IVP
      • Arteriogram
   d. No concurrent infection
   e. No hereditary renal disorders (e.g. polycystic disease)
2. Remove kidney by either anterior or posterior approach with great care to the pedicle, preserving as much ureter as possible with the kidney

Donors – 80% cadaveric

1. Brain stem death
   a. Trauma – 25%
   b. CVA – 40%
   c. Other cause – 35%
2. Contraindications
   a. > 70 years of age
   b. Hypertensive
   c. Diabetes
   d. Systemic infection
   e. Extra-cranial malignant tumour
   f. Renal disease
3. Problems
   a. Diagnostic criteria for brain death
   b. Consent from relatives and coroner (UK), donor card consent
   c. Must be fully ventilated prior to removal of organs
4. Use abdominal approach
   a. Allows removal of both kidneys en bloc with cava and aorta
   b. Allows removal of other organs (liver, pancreas)

Recipient

1. Compatibility
   a. HLA
   b. ABO
   c. Mixed lymphocyte culture
2. Investigations
   a. Gastroscopy – co-existing peptic ulcer
   b. MSU and treat urinary tract infection
3. Correct

   a. Hypertension
   b. Secondary hyperparathyroidism
   c. Osteomalacia
   d. Hypersplenism
4. Consider recipient nephrectomy
   a. Hypertensive chronic renal failure
   b. Polycystic disease, to make room
   c. Chronic pyelonephritis

Transplant operation
1. Cold kidney time – up to 72 hours
2. General anaesthesia with endotracheal intubation

Incision
Extended grid iron (Rutherford–Morrison) in the opposite iliac
fossa to the donor side

Procedure
1. Place donor kidney extra peritoneally
2. Anastomose
   a. Renal artery to internal iliac artery end-to-end
   b. (20% have double artery so use a cuff of aorta for
      anastomosis to external iliac artery)
   c. Renal vein to external iliac vein end-to-side
   d. Ureter to bladder

Postoperative management
1. Immunosuppression
   a. Azathioprine
   b. Corticosteroids
   c. Anti-lymphocyte globulin
   d. Cyclosporin
2. Monitor
   a. Urine output and osmolality (encourage diuresis to diminish
      the chances of acute tubular necrosis)
   b. ECG
   c. Serum potassium
   d. CVP
   e. Beware wound haematoma

Complications
1. Early
   a. Oliguria/anuria
      • Radioisotope renogram
      • IVP
      • Renal angiography
      • Biopsy graft

  b. Renal artery stenosis/leakage
  c. Ureteric stenosis/leakage
  d. Infection
     • Urine   ⎫ Viral
     • Wound   ⎬ Fungal
     • Graft   ⎭ Protozoal
     • Septicaemia
2. Late
  a. Immunosuppression
     • Opportunistic infection
     • Lymphoma
  b. Tertiary hyperparathyroidism

Rejection
1. Hyperacute
  a. Within hours
  b. Due to platelet occlusion as a result of prior
     sensitisation
2. Acute
  a. Up to 6 months
  b. Cell mediated
3. Chronic
  a. 12–18 months
  b. Occlusion due to arteriolar intimal thickening

Assessment of rejection
1. Clinically
  a. Tender graft
  b. Malaise with pyrexia
2. Decreased renal function
  a. Decreased output
  b. Acute renal failure with rising creatinine (>10% change is
     significant)
3. Isotope renogram
4. Percutaneous biopsy or aspiration cytology

Results
1. Operative mortality – 4%
  a. Infection
  b. GI haemorrhage
  c. CVA
  d. Myocardial infarction
2. Graft survival

	1 year	5 years
Related donor	90%	80%
Cadaveric donor	80%	60%

PRINCIPLES OF URINARY DIVERSION

Classify
1. Temporary
2. Permanent

Indications
1. Distal obstruction
2. Incurable fistula
3. Cystectomy
4. Loss of external sphincter
5. Ectopia vesicae
6. Calculi

Problems with diversion
1. Urine collection
2. Ascending urinary infection
3. Reflux
4. Anastomotic stricture
5. Solute reabsorption
6. Carcinogenic effect of solutes

METHODS

Nephrostomy
1. Temporary } Use a Malecot open percutaneous catheter
2. Permanent }

Pyelostomy
1. Catheter
2. Loop

Ureterostomy
Temporary catheterisation
1. From above
2. Retrograde
Permanent
1. Unilateral ureteric disease
   a. High pathology
      • Uretero-ureterostomy
      • Ileal loop interposition
      • Autotransplant kidney to iliac fossa
   b. Low pathology
      • Ureteric bladder reimplantation
      • Boari flap
      • Psoas bladder hitch
2. Bilateral (following cystectomy)
   a. Uretero-cutaneous anastomosis (high incidence of stomal stricture)
   b. Ileal conduit

    c. Colonic implantation (ascending infection, hyperchloraemic acidosis and increased incidence of carcinoma of the distal colon)

    d. Lowsley's operation (rectal bladder)

Bladder

1. Suprapubic catheterisation
2. Urethral catheterisation
3. Urethrotomy

CYSTECTOMY AND ILEAL CONDUIT

Plan of treatment for transitional carcinoma of the bladder

1. T1 carcinoma
    a. Endoscopic resection – review
    b. Multiple recurrent tumours – consider intravesical chemotherapy (Adriamycin, mitomycin, thiotepa, Epodyl)
2. T2 carcinoma
    Endoscopic resection – review, if recurs as T2 then proceed to radiotherapy as for T3
3. T3 carcinoma
    a. 5 500 CGy radiotherapy to the tumour in fractions then either
    b. Review, if recurs then cystectomy
    c. Proceed to cystectomy at completion of radiotherapy
4. T4 carcinoma
    5500 CGy radiotherapy to palliate symptoms with urinary diversion ± cystectomy

Preoperative management

1. Examine the patient standing, sitting and lying flat to find a suitable point in the right iliac fossa to site the ileal conduit
2. Investigations
    a. IVU
    b. Cystoscopy with biopsy and bimanual examination
    c. Pelvic CT scan/pelvic ultrasound
    d. Pelvic lymphangiogram
    e. Distant metastases
      • Chest X-ray
      • Liver ultrasound/isotope scan
      • Skeletal survey/isotope bone scan
3. Antibiotics – broad spectrum with metronidazole prophylaxis
4. Bowel preparation (see p. 104)
5. IVI
6. Nasogastric tube

Pre-incision

1. General anaesthesia with endotracheal intubation
2. Position – supine with steep Trendelenburg tilt
3. Skin preparation of all of abdomen and external genitalia, including vagina

Incision
Mid-line commencing just above symphysis

Procedure
1. Full laparotomy
   a. Exclude intra-abdominal metastases
   b. Assess tumour fixity and operability
2. Expose and dissect out each ureter from the level of the bifurcation of the common iliac arteries downwards, divide the ureters at this level ligating the distal ends, mobilising the proximal ends
3. Ligate both internal iliac arteries in continuity (except in arteriopaths when this may compromise the leg circulation)
4. Mobilise the bladder from the symphysis by blunt dissection of the retropubic space
5. Laterally
   a. Divide the vas in the male
   b. Mobilise and divide the ovarian and uterine pedicles in the female
   c. Clamp, divide and ligate the vesical pedicles containing the superior and inferior vesical vessels
6. Male
   a. Bluntly dissect down around the prostate to separate the urethra and rectum
   b. Lifting the bladder and prostate upwards, clamp and divide the urethra
   c. Peel the prostate and vesicles off the rectum, divide the lateral peritoneal attachment of the bladder and remove the specimen
7. Female
   a. Bluntly dissect the retropubic space, lifting the bladder to palpate the urethra. Divide the urethra as distally as possible
   b. Open the inferior anterior wall of the vagina transversely and divide each lateral wall up to the cervix
   c. Divide the lateral vesical and uterine attachments to deliver the bladder, uterus, ovaries and anterior wall of the vagina en bloc
   d. Close the vagina
8. Dissect out all the pelvic lymph nodes bilaterally for histology
   a. Obturator nodes
   b. Internal iliac chain
   c. Common iliac chain
9. Pack the pelvis to reduce bleeding during the fashioning of the ileal conduit

Ileal conduit
1. Select a loop of distal ileum 20 cm in length commencing about 50 cm from the ileocaecal junction

2. Isolate this loop and anastomose the two ends of the bowel with the loop lying below the mesentery
3. Carefully mobilise the mesentery, avoid damage to the vascular arcades supplying both the loop and the remaining bowel
4. Slit the distal free ends of the ureters for 2 cm and anastomose the splayed ends in a single layer of absorbable suture
5. Pass ureteric catheters up each ureter and into the proximal end of the ileal loop. Pass these catheters the whole length of the conduit
6. Anastomose the ureters to the proximal end of the ileal conduit in a single layer of absorbable suture
7. Complete the conduit by bringing out the distal ileal loop as a spout at the predetermined site in the right iliac fossa

Closure
1. Withdraw the pelvic pack and replace with a Foley balloon catheter passed per urethra, haemostasis is assisted by the balloon being fully inflated and placed on traction
2. Drain the pelvis
3. Close in layers

Postoperative management
1. Remove
   a. Pelvic urethral catheter at 24–48 hours
   b. Pelvic drain when drainage is minimal
   c. Ureteric catheters at 4–5 days
2. Investigations
   Histological examination of specimen and pelvic lymph nodes

Complications
1. Early
   a. Haemorrhage from pelvic veins
   b. Rectal perforation (should be repaired and defunctioning colostomy)
   c. Infection
      • Urinary tract
      • Pelvic abscess
      • Septicaemia
   d. Ileus/obstruction with adhesions
2. Late
   a. Stricture at uretero-ileal anastomosis
   b. Tumour recurrence
   c. Strangulation of ileal conduit
      • Volvulus
      • Prolapse

Prognostic factors
1. Stage of tumour (TNM)
2. Histological grade
3. Tumour size

Prognosis
5 years survival
  a. T1 – >70%
  b. T2 – 50%
  c. T3 – 20%
  d. T4 – 0%

CIRCUMCISION

Indications
1. Religious/social
2. Phimosis
3. Recurrent balanitis (especially diabetics)
4. Prelude to radiotherapy for carcinoma of the penis

Pre-incision
1. General anaesthetic, optional caudal block reduces postoperative pain
2. Position – supine
3. Skin preparation of all of external genitalia, in childhood phimosis gently break down the preputial adhesions with a probe, retract the foreskin and clean the glans

Procedure
1. Apply two straight artery forceps side by side along the midline of the dorsum of the foreskin
2. Incise between these two forceps with scissors to within 0.5 cm of the corona
3. Continue this incision circumferentially around the foreskin in both directions. Pick up any bleeding vessels in artery forceps
4. Beware retraction of bleeding vessels
5. Do not use monopolar diathermy on the penis
6. The two incisions meet at the frenulum – place a clip across this and excise the foreskin distal to this
7. Transfix the frenulum with an absorbable suture
8. Ligate the vessels with absorbable sutures
9. Suture the two layers of the foreskin with several interrupted absorbable sutures
10. Dress loosely

Complications
1. Infants may go into retention with pain

2. After dissection of extensive prepucial adhesions, there may be considerable ulceration of the glans which may result in meatal stenosis

DARTOS POUCH ORCHIDOPEXY FOR UNDESCENDED/ECTOPIC TESTIS

Reasons for surgery
1. 90% have associated inguinal hernia
2. May improve spermatogenesis
3. Reduces risk of torsion (which is greater for undescended and ectopic testes)
4. Cosmetic/psychological
5. Does not reduce the increased risk of malignant change in the testis but does render such change more immediately obvious to the patient
6. Optimal time to operate before 2 years old
7. If impalpable – localise with ultrasound/CT
8. If bilateral undescended testes – exclude anorchism by measuring the serum testosterone response to an injection of HCG (no response = anorchic)

Preoperative management
Examine the patient
    a. Exclude retractile testis
    b. Mark the side

Pre-incision
1. General anaesthetic
2. Position – supine
3. Skin preparation of all of genitalia and groin on relevant side

Incision
Groin skin crease

Procedure
1. Open inguinal canal by dividing external oblique aponeurosis from the external ring and locate the testes
  a. 90% of undescended testes lie within the inguinal canal
  b. 80% of ectopic testes lie in the superficial inguinal pouch
2. Carefully open the layers of the cord and dissect out the indirect inguinal hernia
3. Perform a herniotomy (*see* Inguinal hernia repair, p. 14)
4. Gently separate all the fibres of cremaster from the components of the cord until the vas and vessels lie free, thus lengthening these structures without tension
5. Dartos pouch
    a. Insert the left index finger into the scrotum from above

    b. Make a 1 cm incision into the skin of the scrotum and pass artery forceps through the dartos layer up to the groin, grasp the mobilised testis and bring down to lie between the dartos and skin of the scrotum

Closure
1. No drains
2. Close in layers

Postoperative management
Most children can go home the same evening

Complications
1. Small atrophic testis at operation – excise
2. Failed reduction – gain as much length with the first operation then subsequently re-explore and mobilise into scrotum
3. Early – testicular infarction with cord damage
4. Late – malignant change (×20–30 incidence of malignancy of normal testis)
5. If reduction fails or the testis lost, the optimal age for a testicular prosthesis implant is 15 years

HYDROCELE – LORD'S OPERATION

Preoperative management
1. Children – manage as inguinal hernia (*see* p. 14)
2. Adult
    a. Careful history and examination – mark the side
    b. Exclude
       • Testicular tumour
       • Trauma
       • Epididymo-orchitis
    c. If bilateral – exclude ascites
    d. Aspirate
       Culture
       Cytology
       Always examine testis after aspiration

Pre-incision
1. General or local anaesthetic
2. Position – supine
3. Skin preparation of all of external genitalia

Incision
Transversely across the hemiscrotum through all layers including the hydrocele sac

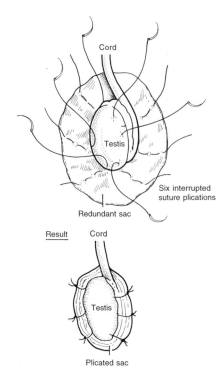

Fig. 24 Lord's procedure.

Procedure (Fig. 24)

1. Control bleeding from cut edges and suck out hydrocele fluid
2. Place 3 interrupted sutures each side of the testis, commencing at the edge of the sac, picking up several bites of the sac and finishing on the tunica at the junction of testis and epididymis
3. When all 6 sutures are in place, tighten them up to plicate the sac, obliterating the hydrocele and tie them
4. Ensure absolute haemostasis
5. No drains
6. Close in layers

Postoperative management

Apply a scrotal support for comfort

Complications

Scrotal haematoma

EXCISION OF VARICOCELE

Preoperative management
1. Investigations
   a. If for infertility – sperm count and analysis
   b. IVP/US for left sided varicocele has a pick up rate for renal carcinoma of < 1%
2. Examine and mark the side with the patient standing

Pre-incision
1. General anaesthetic
2. Position – supine
3. Skin preparation of groin

Incision
Groin skin crease

Procedure
1. Open inguinal canal by dividing external oblique aponeurosis from the external ring
2. Open the layers of the cord to display the distended pampiniform plexus/testicular vein branches
3. Dissect out all the pampiniform plexus, ligate and divide all these veins

Closure
1. Meticulous haemostasis
2. No drains
3. Close in layers

Postoperative management
Investigations
   • Infertility
   • Testicular biopsy
   • Serial sperm analyses

Complications
1. Early
   a. Scrotal haemotoma
   b. Damage to cord
      • Vas
      • Vessels
2. Late
   Recurrent varicocele

ORCHIDECTOMY FOR TESTICULAR TUMOUR

Preoperative management

1. Informed consent for orchidectomy, examine and mark the side
2. Consider pretreatment sperm banking
3. Investigations
   a. Ultrasound/CT
      - Primary tumour
      - Para-aortic nodes
      - Liver
   b. Chest X-ray and CT
   c. Lymphangiography of para-aortic nodes
   d. Isotope bone scan
   e. Blood for tumour markers
      - Alphafetoprotein
      - CEA
      - Beta-human chorionic gonadotrophin elevated in teratoma

Pre-incision

1. General anaesthetic
2. Position – supine
3. Skin preparation of groin region

Incision

Groin skin crease

Procedure

1. Open the inguinal canal by dividing the external oblique aponeurosis commencing from the external ring
2. Mobilise the cord within the canal and cross clamp it
3. Divide the cord and ligate the two ends with non-absorbable ligatures
4. Deliver the testis by traction to the distal cord, thus inverting the scrotum, ligate and divide the gubernaculum
5. Send the specimen for histological examination

Closure

No drains and close in layers, apply a scrotal support for comfort

Postoperative investigations

   a. Histological examination of the tumour
   b. Serial investigations for tumour markers since metastases may now become biochemically apparent

Complications

Scrotal haematoma

Vascular surgery

PRINCIPLES OF ELECTIVE VASCULAR RECONSTRUCTION
1. Never risk life to save a limb
2. Full preoperative workup must establish nature and extent of disease, showing a good run-off

Indications
1. Severe claudication < 200 m
2. A sudden recent deterioration
3. Pathology is above the knee
4. Claudication distance less than angina distance

Contraindications
1. Severe angina
2. Systemic malignancy
3. Recent myocardial infarction
4. Pathology is below knee (poor run-off) except in limb salvage for critical ischaemia

Relative contraindications
Continuing smoking

Indications for amputation
1. Gangrene
2. Severe rest pain not amenable to arterial reconstruction
3. Uncontrollable infection, especially in diabetics
4. Malignancy in limb not amenable to more conservative treatment

Types of surgery
1. Arterial
   a. Endarterectomy
   b. Profundoplasty
   c. Bypass graft
      • Reverse or in situ vein
      • Synthetic

    d. Angioplasty
- Dotter and Gruntzig percutaneous balloon (radiological)
- Vein patch
- Synthetic patch (dacron, Goretex, etc.)

2. Sympathectomy
    a. Surgical
    b. Chemical

3. Endarterectomy
    a. Only for larger arteries which do not cross joints (e.g. aorta, iliacs and carotids)
    b. Problems
- Subsequent intimal deposition 1–2 mm thick
- Distal intimal dissection
- Extent of disease

4. Vein (bypass graft/patch)
    a. Best material, available from long saphenous or cephalic veins
    b. Undergoes changes
- Narrows with subendothelial hypertrophy and intimal clot deposition
- 10% develop atheroma
- Anastomotic stenosis
- Fibrosis develops at valves and tributaries

5. Synthetic
    a. Dacron
- Very good replacement for large vessels (> 10 mm)
Problems
- Tend to buckle across joints
- False aneurysms at anastomoses
- Thick intimal deposition (2–4 mm)
- Infection of implanted foreign material
    b. PTFE (Goretex)
- Useful for smaller arteries (e.g. superficial femoral)
- Easy to suture and requires no pre-clotting
Problems
- High 3-year failure rate (> 30%) compared with vein infection
- Tendency to kink

Technical principles

1. Aim for a smooth flow by
    a. Avoiding loose flaps
    b. Avoiding both intrinsic and extrinsic constriction
    c. Avoid narrowing at anastomoses

2. Handle all arteries and grafts with care

3. Strict asepsis

4. Preoperative antisepsis

5. Per and postoperative antibiotics
6. Peroperative anticoagulation with heparin

Operations for aorta-iliac disease
1. Aorto-iliac endarterectomy
2. Aorto-femoral synthetic Dacron graft
3. Femoro-femoral Dacron graft
4. Axillo-femoral subcutaneous Dacron graft

Operations for femoropopliteal disease
1. Femoropopliteal bypass
   a. Reverse saphenous vein
   b. In situ saphenous veins
   c. PTFE (Goretex)
2. Superficial femoral endarterectomy
3. Profundoplasty

Operations for internal carotid disease
1. Endarterectomy
2. Extracranial (superficial temporal) to intracranial (middle cerebral) anastomosis

Operations for coronary artery disease
1. Aorto-coronary artery vein bypass graft
2. Endarterectomy (short lesion in large artery)
3. Internal mammary coronary anastomosis

AORTO-BIFEMORAL BYPASS GRAFT
Indications
1. Severe aorto-iliac atherosclerosis
2. Leriche syndrome

Preoperative preparation
1. Investigations to establish extent of disease
   a. Doppler pressure studies
   b. Arteriography
2. Manage concomitant problems
   a. Stop smoking
   b. Control diabetes
   c. Control hypertension
3. Antiseptic bath prior to surgery with swabs sent from the patient's skin and orifices to exclude foci of pathogenic organisms (especially *Staphylococcus aureus*)
4. Antibiotic prophylaxis
   a. Flucloxacillin or cephalosporin for 2–5 days
5. Tubes
   a. Catheterise, nasogastric tube and intravenous infusion
   b. Arterial line optional

Pre-incision
1. General anaesthesia with endotracheal intubation
2. Position – supine with arms by the side
3. Skin preparation from mid thorax to knees
4. Incisions
   a. Longitudinal incisions over each common femoral artery at the groin (12 cm in length)
   b. Transverse abdominal (healing is better and is less painful than a longitudinal incision)

Procedures
1. Assess patency of groin arteries
2. Dissect out both common femoral arteries as they pass under the inguinal ligament to beyond their bifurcation
3. Beware
   a. Femoral vein, medially
   b. Femoral nerve, laterally
   c. Avoid damage to groin lymph nodes
4. Place silastic slings to control the common femoral, superficial femoral and profunda femoris arteries; smaller branches may also need slings
5. Full laparotomy to exclude other pathology
6. Pack off small bowel
7. Incise peritoneum to the left of the small bowel mesentery to approach the aorta
8. Expose the aorta from the level of the left renal vein down to the bifurcation taking care to avoid and protect the inferior mesenteric artery
9. Beware
   a. The vena cava on the right of the aorta
   b. The left common iliac vein behind the aortic bifurcation
10. Slings around the aorta at the upper and lower levels of dissection are optional (it may be necessary to mobilise both common iliac arteries and control these with slings if the aortic segment is short)
11. Create tunnels behind the inguinal ligaments by blunt dissection
12. Withdraw 20 ml of blood and preclot the graft if necessary
13. Heparinise the patient with 5000 units either intravenously or directly into the aorta. Wait three minutes
14. Now clamp across the aorta proximally and distally
15. Clamp the common femoral arteries with appropriate clamps and their branches with bull-dog clamps
16. Control lumbar arteries either from without or within by suture
17. Open the aorta on its anterior surface; this may now require a local endarterectomy

18. Cut the bifurcation graft to correct length with prebifurcation segment as short as possible to improve the haemodynamics of flow
19. Suture graft to aortic arteriotomy with continuous 3/0 prolene (either end-to-side or by aortic transection and end-to-end) and test the anastomosis by releasing the aortic clamp
20. Clamp the proximal graft and release the aortic clamps
21. Pass sponge forceps from each groin wound through the pre-dissected tunnels and withdraw the limbs of the graft to the groin wounds
22. Open both common femoral arteries on their anterior surfaces just above their bifurcation. Avoid local endarterectomies
23. Anastomose one limb of the graft to the common femoral arteriotomies with 4/0 continuous prolene. The graft may be used as a patch to widen the orifice of the profunda
24. Release the clamps in turn to evacuate any clot which may have formed via the blow holes
25. Establish flow in the completed limb
26. Suck out all the blood from the second limb and complete the second anastomosis
27. Release all the clamps and recheck the anastomoses

Closure
1. Once the ooze of blood from the graft and the anastomotic suture lines have subsided (heparin may occasionally require reversal with protamine) then commence closure
2. No abdominal drains but suction drains to both groins
3. Close the peritoneum over the graft in the abdomen to make it completely retroperitoneal and close the abdomen in layers
4. Close the groin in layers

Postoperative management
1. Monitor peripheral pulses continuously and measure the arterial pressures in both legs by Doppler
2. Continue antibiotics for 5 days

Complications
1. Early
   a. Anastomotic leakage uncommon
   b. Graft thrombosis is rare, needs re-exploration and thrombectomy (if this occurs there is usually poor run-in or run-off which must be dealt with)
   c. Graft infection
   d. Small bowel obstruction with adhesions to exposed graft if peritoneal cover is incomplete
   e. Lymphatic groin fistulae, usually heal spontaneously
2. Late
   a. Aorto-enteric fistula
   b. Recurrent atheroma

REVERSE SAPHENOUS VEIN FEMOROPOPLITEAL BYPASS GRAFT

Indications
Severe arterial insufficiency of the lower leg due to occlusion of the superficial femoral artery with poor collateral circulation between the profunda femoris and popliteal arteries

Preoperative preparation
1. Examine and mark out the vein with the patient standing
2. Investigations to establish extent of disease
   a. Doppler pressure studies at rest and after exercise
   b. Arteriography
3. Manage concomitant problems
   a. Stop smoking
   b. Control diabetes
   c. Control hypertension
4. Antisepsis
   a. Shave the leg and antiseptic baths prior to surgery
   b. Preoperative and peroperative antibiotic prophylaxis with flucloxacillin continued for 2–5 days
   c. Mark out long saphenous vein with patient standing
5. IVI

Pre-incision
1. Either spinal or general anaesthesia with optional endotracheal intubation
2. Position – supine with leg slightly flexed and abducted at the hip and the knee slightly flexed. Avoid compression of lateral popliteal nerve
3. Skin preparation above groin to above ankle, whole leg
4. Towel up to expose leg and place foot in a clear sterile bowel bag

Incision
Groin incision 12 cm in length longitudinally over common femoral artery and a separate incision commencing distal to this over the length of the long saphenous vein to below the knee. The skin bridge between these two incisions improves lymphatic drainage from the leg

Procedure
1. Groin operator (Fig. 25)
   a. Dissect out the common femoral artery and its branches at the bifurcation. Place slings around the common femoral, profunda femoris and superficial femoral arteries (other larger branches if necessary)
   b. Dissect out the termination of long saphenous vein as it enters the femoral vein, ligate all its tributaries and its

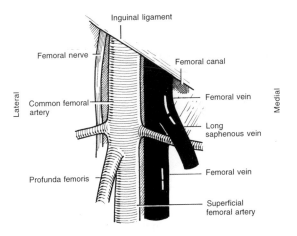

Fig. 25   Anatomy of the femoral artery.

termination at the femoral vein. Divide the long saphenous vein 1–2 cm from its termination
   c. Dissect out the saphenous vein distally ligating and dividing all its branches as it passes under the skin bridge
2. Lower operator
   a. Dissect out the lower popliteal artery dividing the deep fascia behind the saphenous vein, just below the knee
   b. Displace sartorius posteriorly or divide it near its insertion
   c. Bluntly dissect out the neurovascular bundle in the popliteal space as it passes between the heads of gastrocnemius (the medial head may be divided to improve access)
   d. Isolate the artery as it passes from medial to lateral behind the popliteal vein which is receiving the short saphenous vein, the tibial nerve lies laterally in the neurovascular bundle
   e. Place slings around the artery to control it
   f. Dissect out the long saphenous vein for the length of the incision, ligating and dividing all its tributaries. If the vein is inadequate, then use synthetic graft (e.g. PTFE)
   g. Now remove the long saphenous vein and turn it round, gently, inflate it with heparinised saline to test for leaks from tears and missed tributaries which must be closed
   h. Heparinise the patient with 5000 units either intravenously or into the common femoral artery. Wait 3 minutes
   i. Clamp and control the femoral and popliteal arteries and all their local branches
   j. Open both arteries and if necessary perform a local endarterectomy of the common femoral artery

k. Replace the reversed vein subcutaneously and anastomose it firstly to the common femoral artery with a 5/0 prolene continuous suture side-to-end

l. Now anastomose the lower end of the vein graft to the popliteal artery end-to-side with a similar suture material, leaving a small blow-hole

m. Test the upper anastomosis by flushing through and out of the blow hole at the lower anastomosis. Allow any thrombus in the distal arteries out of the blow hole by backwards (retrograde) flow. Close the artery and remove the controlling clamps

Closure

1. Once the anastomotic suture line ooze has ceased and graft patency is established commence closure
2. Place suction drains in groin wound and popliteal fossa
3. Close deep fascia and skin separately

Postoperative management

1. Check pedal arterial pressures by Doppler regularly during recovery
2. Nurse with leg slightly flexed at the knee and supported for 48 hours, mobilise after this
3. Antibiotic cover for 48 hours

Complications

1. Graft occlusion
   a. Early
      - Usually due to technical error in surgery (can be reduced by peroperative angiography)
   b. Late
      - Recurrent disease either above, below or in graft, especially with continuing smoking
2. Lymphatic leakage at groin
3. Infection less serious with vein graft but increases the risk of secondary haemorrhage

PROFUNDOPLASTY

Indications

1. Thigh claudication due to profunda stenosis
2. Lower leg ischaemia with profunda popliteal collateral circulation

Preoperative preparation (Fig. 25)

1. As for femoropopliteal bypass (see p. 162)
2. Investigations
   Lateral or oblique femoral arteriogram

Pre-incision
As for femoropopliteal bypass (which may be necessary should profundoplasty not be feasible)

Incision
Longitudinally for 12 cm over femoral pulse at groin

Procedure
1. Dissect out common femoral, superficial femoral and profunda femoris arteries in the femoral triangle
2. Trace the profunda distally, ligating and dividing veins as they cross it, isolating its branches with slings
3. Isolate and remove 5–6 cm of superficial vein. It is preferable to preserve the long saphenous vein for further arterial reconstruction
4. Place slings around all the major arteries and heparinise the patient with 5000 units intravenously. Wait 5 minutes and clamp the major vessels at the edge of the operative field
5. Perform a long arteriotomy, commencing on the mid and common femoral artery, passing down the profunda and finishing at its bifurcation or beyond if the vessel is still abnormal
6. Perform a local endarterectomy for the length of the arteriotomy, suturing down the distal flaps of atheroma with non-absorbable sutures
7. Close the arteriotomy with a long reversed vein patch
8. Remove clamps to establish and check flow, await haemostasis at suture line

Closure
1. Suction drain to deep wound
2. Close in layers

Postoperative management
As for femoropopliteal bypass (see p. 162) but can mobilise earlier

CAROTID ENDARTERECTOMY

Indications
1. Carotid stenosis with
   a. Unilateral transient ischaemic attacks or amaurosis fugax
   b. Mild persistent cerebrovascular defect

Relative indications
Severe carotid stenosis (> 90%) without neurological deficit

Contraindications
1. Recent major stroke
2. Asymptomatic carotid bruit with less than 75% stenosis
3. Severely symptomatic abdominal aortic aneurysm
4. Disseminated malignant disease

Relative contraindications
Second side operation within 2 weeks of first side

Preoperative management
1. Investigation to establish diagnosis
   a. Duplex Doppler studies of carotids
   b. Arteriography
   c. CT scan of brain
2. Aspirin is optional
3. Examine and mark the side

Pre-incision
1. Position – supine with shoulders elevated on a pad to extend the neck and head turned away
2. Peroperative ECG
3. Intravenous line and radial arterial line for continuous arterial pressure monitoring
4. Skin preparation from neck to thorax
5. Drapes, expose from parotid area to root of neck

Incision
Along anterior border of sternomastoid centring on the carotid bifurcation

Procedure
1. Divide platysma with the skin
2. Retract greater auricular nerve posteriorly in upper part of wound and divide the deep fascia in the line of the incision
3. Place a self retaining retractor to hold sternomastoid posteriorly, mobilise, ligate and divide the common facial vein to expose the carotid sheath
4. Dissect the tissues of the carotid sheath off the carotids, exposing and preserving the hypoglossal nerve as it crosses the two carotids above the bifurcation of the common carotid artery
5. Beware descendens hypoglossi and vagus nerve
6. Gently retract the hypoglossal nerve and descendens hypoglossi away from the arteries
7. Gently pass slings around the common carotid, internal carotid and external carotid arteries
8. Beware rough handling causing embolisation of atheroma
9. Heparinise with 5000 units and wait 3 minutes

10. Now gently occlude the carotids and start the stop watch which records carotid occlusion time, mobilise the common carotid bifurcation, clamping all major branches
11. Measure the internal carotid stump pressure to determine whether a shunt is necessary
12. A shunt is necessary if the internal carotid pressure is less than one-third of the radial artery pressure
13. Perform an arteriotomy at the site of the occlusion and if necessary pass a Javid shunt above and below the occlusion. Perform the endarterectomy
14. Close the arteriotomy with 6/0 Prolene, removing the shunt at the end
15. Remove the clamps, first the external, then the common and finally the internal carotid, noting the clamped time on the stop watch
16. Await haemostasis from suture line

Closure
1. Haemostasis, swab and instrument check
2. Place suction drain in the wound
3. Close in layers, deep fascia, and skin

Postoperative management
Nurse in intensive care unit with quarter hourly observation of pulse, blood pressure and neurological observations.

Complications
1. Stroke (early) 2%, may be precipitated by hypotension
2. Mortality < 2%

CERVICAL SYMPATHECTOMY – SUPRACLAVICULAR APPROACH

Indications
1. Hyperhydrosis of hand
2. Raynaud's phenomenon
   a. Buerger's
   b. Polio
   c. Syringomyelia
3. Little use in Raynaud's disease

Preoperative preparation
1. Mark the side
2. Warn the patient about the risk of Horner's syndrome and exclude pre-existing Horner's

Pre-incision
1. General anaesthesia with endotracheal intubation
2. Position – supine with a sandbag under the shoulders and neck extended with head turned away

Incision
8 cm long, 2 cm above and parallel to mid-third of clavicle

Procedure
1. Divide
   a. External jugular vein (beware air embolism)
   b. Lateral border of sternomastoid
   c. Omohyoid central tendon – marking the ends with ligatures
   d. Lateral scalenus anterior
2. Beware phrenic nerve on scalenus anterior
3. Beware subclavian vein inferiorly, and thoracic duct on left (if this is divided inadvertently, then ligate both free ends)
4. Insert torch on stick
5. Place a sling around the subclavian artery, retracting it downwards
6. Beware brachial plexus posteriorly
7. Divide Sibson's fascia, depressing the dome of the diaphragm to palpate stellate ganglion on neck of first rib
8. Feel for and visualise the second and third thoracic sympathetic ganglia, which are to be removed
9. Remove these ganglia. Send the specimen for confirmatory histology
10. Beware opening pleura

Closure
1. If the pleura is inadvertently opened, reinflate the lung with positive pressure ventilation before closing
2. Suction drain in the floor of the wound
3. Repair
   a. Omohyoid
   b. Sternomastoid
4. Close in layers

Postoperative care
1. Nurse sitting upright
2. Investigation
   a. Chest X-ray in recovery, exclude pneumothorax
   b. Histology of ganglia to confirm procedure
3. Complications
   a. Horner's syndrome with T1/stellate ganglion damage
   b. Pneumothorax
   c. Thoracic duct fistula, especially if damage to the thoracic duct is unrecognised at the time of surgery

PRINCIPLES OF SURGICAL LUMBAR SYMPATHECTOMY

Indications
Small vessel disease of the feet

Preoperative preparation
1. If diabetic, test vibration sensations in the feet, since if absent, indicates that autonomic neuropathy also exists therefore sympathectomy little use
2. NG tube especially if bilateral since postoperative ileus is common

Pre-incision
1. General anaesthesia with endotracheal intubation
2. Position – supine with a sandbag under the lumbar region on the appropriate side
3. Skin preparation of all of abdomen

Incision
Transverse, lateral to umbilicus

Procedure
1. Deepen the incision through muscle layers with cutting diathermy as far as the peritoneum, keep outside peritoneum
2. Mobilise posteriorly between peritoneum and transversus abdominis and gently work over psoas to its medial side
3. Pack off retroperitoneal space with packs placed superiorly, inferiorly and medially, retracting the peritoneum and its contents medially with a large retractor
4. Beware
   a. Ureter
   b. Gonadal vessels
   c. Aorta on left   } All travelling vertically
   d. IVC on right
   e. Genitofemoral nerve
   f. Lumbar vessels
   g. Para-aortic lymph nodes (since they resemble sympathetic ganglia)
5. Identify sympathetic chain lying in groove between psoas and lumbar vertebral bodies visually and by palpation
6. Lift chain with nerve hook and remove the second and third lumbar ganglia. Send for histological confirmation

Closure
Close in layers

Postoperative management
Complications
    a. Retroperitoneal haematoma
    b. Ileus especially if bilateral sympathetectomy
    c. Pain in distribution of the genitofemoral nerve

BELOW-KNEE AMPUTATION FOR ISCHAEMIA
Preoperative management
1. Examine and mark the side
2. Special tests
    Is the case not suitable for arterial reconstruction?
    a. Dopplers
    b. Arteriogram
3. Antibiotic
    a. Benzyl penicillin
    b. Metronidazole

Pre-incision
1. General or spinal anaesthesia
2. No tourniquet
3. Skin preparation
    a. Ankle to low abdomen (therefore possible to proceed to
    above-knee amputation if necessary)
    b. Mark out skin flaps anterior
      • 10 cm below tibial condyle, posterior
      • 20 cm below tibial condyle

Incision (Fig. 26)
Along line of skin flaps to deep fascia, ligate superficial
veins

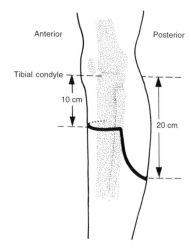

Fig. 26 Incision for below-knee amputation.

Procedure
1. Assess bleeding from skin edges. If poor, then probably not viable and consider above-knee amputation
2. Deepen incision in the anterior compartment dividing its muscles: tibialis anterior, extensor hallucis longus and extensor digitorum longus, ligate and divide the anterior tibial vessels
3. Divide the tibia transversely at the level of the anterior flap and cut out an anterior bevel which should be filled until absolutely smooth and rounded and the filings washed out
4. Divide the fibula with a Gigli saw 1–2 cm above the level of the division of the tibia
5. Divide the peroneal muscles at the same level as the fibula, ligating the peroneal vessels
6. Ligate and divide the posterior tibial vessels then, with a sharp knife, divide the muscles of the deep compartment (tibialis posterior, flexor, digitorum longus and flexor hallucis longus) and the posterior compartment (soleus and gastrocnemius) between the posterior edge of the tibia and the posterior skin flap, ligating the deep veins of the calf
7. Shave down the muscle of the posterior flap so that it lies comfortably opposing the anterior flap

Closure
1. Haemostasis must be meticulous
    a. Use ligatures
    b. Avoid diathermy
2. Suction drain to raw muscle bed
3. Suture
    a. Deep fascia of posterior flap to deep fascia and periosteum of anterior flap with an absorbable suture
    b. Skin, interrupted monofilament sutures of Steri strips®
4. Dress the stump
    a. Gauze
    b. Cotton wool
    c. Netalast

Postoperative management
1. Avoid any pressure, traditional stump bandaging is dangerous
2. Keep knee in extension to reduce flexion contractures
3. Encourage early exercises, especially with the patient prone for flexion and extension
4. Commence walking training using an inflatable prosthesis
5. Attend fittings for prosthesis once wound healed

Complications
1. Early
    a. Infection (especially *Clostridium welchii*)
    b. Haematoma
    c. Skin flap ischaemia

2. Late
   a. Stump
      - Neuroma
      - Osteoma
   b. Phantom limb (treat with carbamazepine)

ABOVE-KNEE AMPUTATION FOR ISCHAEMIA
Preoperative management
1. Special investigations
   a. Examine to assess level of ischaemia and mark the side
   b. Arterial Doppler pressures
   c. Arteriography
2. Prophylaxis for *Clostridia* and coliforms for anus
   a. Penicillin
   b. Metronidazole

Pre-incision
1. General or spinal anaesthesia
   a. No tourniquet
2. Skin preparation
   a. Low abdomen to upper shin with upper thigh to knee exposed
   b. Elevate knee with bowl to gain access posteriorly
   c. Mark out equal anterior and posterior skin flaps with medial and lateral apices 10 cm above the femoral condyles (Fig. 27)

Incision
Along line of skin flaps to deep fascia, ligating superficial veins

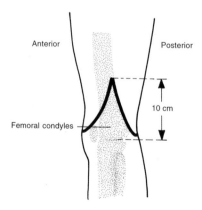

Fig. 27 Skin incision for above-knee amputation.

Procedure
1. Assess skin flap bleeding for viability
2. Deepen anterior flap through quadriceps femoris to femur, (ligate all major muscular vessels)
3. Locate superficial femoral artery and vein in adductor canal – ligate and divide vessels separately
4. Divide
   a. Adductors (magnus and longus)
   b. Sciatic nerve (ligate nutrient artery) and allow to retract
   c. Hamstrings (semimembranosus, semitendinosus and biceps femoris) posteriorly
   d. Ligating all bleeding muscular vessels
5. Place muscle guard on femur 10 cm above femoral condyles and divide femur at this point
6. File femoral edges to remove sharp edges and wash out filings

Closure
1. Absolute haemostasis with ligatures (avoid diathermy)
2. Swabs and instruments
3. Suction drain to deep layers
4. Loosely suture adductors to vastus lateralis over femoral stump
5. Suture superficial quadriceps to hamstrings with loose absorbable sutures
6. Close deep fascia of anterior and posterior flaps
7. Close skin
8. Bandage stump with
   a. Gauze
   b. Cotton wool
   c. Netalast

Postoperative management
1. Avoid traditional stump bandaging which is harmful
2. If supine, place sandbags over stump to prevent flexion deformity with unopposed psoas flexion
3. Commence stump exercises early
4. Arrange limb fitting and mobilisation on stump when wound healed

Complications
1. Early
   a. Infection, especially *Clostridium welchii* and anaerobic coliforms
   b. Skin flap ischaemia
   c. Flexion contraction deformity
2. Late
   a. Phantom limb
   b. Stump
      • Neuroma
      • Osteoma

VARICOSE VEIN SURGERY

Indications
1. Venous ulceration
2. Symptoms of venous stasis (itch, ache)

Contraindications
Post-phlebitic syndrome

Preoperative preparation
1. Assess varicosities
   a. To determine appropriate treatment. 90% of patients have long sapheno-femoral vein incompetence. True short saphenous varicosities are rare
   b. To locate the site of all incompetent superficial to deep communications, especially sapheno-femoral incompetence
   c. Mark the site of all varicosities and incompetent perforating veins (Fig. 28)
2. Investigations
   a. Doppler location of incompetent perforating veins
   b. Venogram, if leg is post-phlebitic

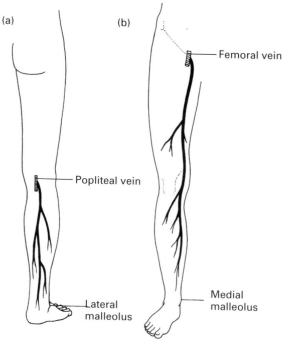

Fig. 28 Marking varicose veins. Route of (a) short saphenous vein; (b) long saphenous vein.

Pre-incision
1. General anaesthesia is preferable to local anaesthesia
2. Position
   a. Anterior veins, supine with legs apart
   b. Posterior veins, prone with legs apart

Incision
1. Groin, 4 cm in length in groin crease medial to femoral pulse
2. Long saphenous strip, 3 cm longitudinally anterior to medial malleolus and groin incision
3. Short saphenous ligation, 3 cm transverse lateral to the midline of the popliteal fossa
4. Perforating veins, 1–2 cm immediately over the site of the incompetent perforating vein
5. Stab avulsions, 2 mm stabs at site of avulsions

Procedure
1. Groin tie
   a. At the groin, dissect out the long saphenous vein as it enters the cribriform fascia, identifying all its tributaries, including the superficial epigastric, superficial pudendal and superficial external iliac veins
   b. Ligate and divide all these tributaries and the long saphenous vein as it enters the femoral vein (failure of surgery is usually due to a branch being missed and subsequently becoming varicose)
2. Stripping
   a. Identify the long saphenous vein at the ankle and dissect out the sapheno-femoral junction as for a groin tie operation
   b. Beware the saphenous nerve lying beside the vein at the ankle
   c. Open the vein at the ankle and pass the stripper proximally negotiating the venous tortuosities to the groin where the stripper head can be attached
   d. Strip the vein from the groin to the ankle. This way reduces the chance of inadvertent damage to the saphenous nerve. Prior to stripping bandage the leg firmly from groin to ankle
3. Short saphenous vein
   Ligate and divide it as it enters the deep fascia of the popliteal fossa (this may need an on-table venogram to determine its junction with the popliteal vein)
4. Incompetent perforating veins
   Dissect out the varicosities over the perforating vein and ligate and divide all the branches, including the perforator as it enters the deep fascia
5. Stab avulsions
   Insert fine mosquito forceps through the stabs to pick up the underlying vein, gently withdrawing it. Apply gently, tractions to avulse the vein and control bleeding with direct pressure

Closure
1. Close skin except stab avulsions which need no closure
2. In every case, bandage the leg fully to the level of the highest vein

Postoperative management
Mobilise as soon as possible in support stockings

LEAKING ABDOMINAL AORTIC ANEURYSM
Always suspect the diagnosis in any elderly patient who presents with sudden onset of abdominal pain and hypotension. These patients have a leaking abdominal aortic aneurysm until proven otherwise

Preoperative preparation
1. Establish diagnosis
   a. Clinically, reinforced by plain X-rays of abdomen including lateral view which may show an eggshell rim of calcification around the aneurysm
   b. Cross-match 8 units immediately
2. Transfer directly to the operating theatre and continue resuscitation in the anaesthetic room
3. Insert
   a. At least two venous lines, including a central venous catheter
   b. Catheter
   c. NG tube
      Arterial line } Can possibly wait until patient anaesthetised
4. Do not waste time trying to get the patient's blood pressure up prior to anaesthesia
5. Antibiotics with induction
   a. Broad spectrum
   b. Flucloxacillin
6. No heparin

Pre-incision
1. Have the following instruments ready prior to making the incision
   a. Aortic compressor to get control of the aorta with compression through the lesser sac
   b. 3 foley urethral catheters with syringes ready to inflate balloons
   c. A selection of large vascular clamps such as
      • Satinsky
      • De Bakey
      • CraaFoord
2. Place the conscious patient on the table, surgeon on the right, paint the abdomen with iodine in alcohol and towel up for a long mid-line incision
3. Induce general anaesthesia and intubate

Procedure
1. On induction perform a long mid-line incision (since the tamponade effect of abdominal muscle tone is now lost)
2. Get control
3. Pack small bowel up to the right
4. Small retroperitoneal leak
   a. Dissect peritoneum off aorta and place clamps across the neck and lower end of the sac
   b. If you lose control during the procedure then incise the sac and push your right thumb up into the neck. Replace it with Foley catheter and inflate the balloon to control bleeding
   c. Place Foley catheters distally into both common iliac arteries and underrun lumbar artery orifices with silk
5. If there is a torrential intraperitoneal haemorrhage, compress the aorta via the lesser sac with an aortic compressor, suck out the peritoneum and then manage as above
6. Structures to beware in all these procedures
   a. Inferior vena cava to the right
   b. Inferior mesenteric vein to the left
   c. Left common iliac vein below aortic bifurcation
   d. Left renal vein at the neck of the sac
7. Proceed
8. Incise sac longitudinally and semi-circumferentially at its neck
9. Underrun orifices of lumbar and median sacral arteries
10. Oversew orifice of the inferior mesenteric artery
11. Clean out organised clot within the sac, select graft
    a. Tube/bifurcation
    b. Size
    c. Knitted versus woven Dacron
12. Insert graft with single continuous layer of monofilament 3/0 Prolene suture, first at top end and then at the lower end
13. Prior to closure of lower end, check for back flow – if this is minimal then Fogarty catheter distally for emboli of fibrin and thrombus
14. Inspect sigmoid colon for ischaemia due to ligation of inferior mesenteric artery
15. Close aneurysm sac over Dacron graft

Closure
1. Haemostasis
2. Repair posterior peritoneum
3. No drains
4. Close peritoneum over graft to prevent adhesions between small bowel and the Dacron
5. Close abdomen in layers

Problems of procedure
1. Distal emboli, needs Fogarty embolectomy
2. Aneurysm extends into iliac arteries then use aorta bifemoral bifurcation graft with ligation of iliac aneurysms

Postoperative care
Nursing
   a. ITU for 24 hours with half-hourly observation, especially
      • Pulse and BP
      • CVP
      • ECG
      • Feet – pulses (by palpation and Doppler)
                  temperature of skin
      • Urine output
   b. Check Hb and transfuse accordingly

Complications
1. Early
   a. Graft anastomosis suture line leakage
   b. Bleeding as blood pressure rises after large transfusion
   c. Acute renal failure
   d. Myocardial infarction
   e. Acute sigmoid colon ischaemia
   f. Emboli to legs (trash foot)
2. Late
   a. Other aneurysms, especially
      • Iliac
      • Femoral
      • Splenic
      • Thoracic aorta
      • Popliteal
   b. False aneurysm of graft especially at suture line
   c. Graft infection
   d. Aorto-duodenal fistula

FEMORAL EMBOLECTOMY
Always suspect in a patient (particularly elderly, in atrial fibrillation, or postmyocardial infarction) who
presents with the sudden onset of a cool, anaesthetic dead leg

Preoperative preparation
1. Mark side

2. If the diagnosis is suspected
   a. Fully heparinise with 10 000 units i.v. as a bolus and continue as an infusion of 10 000 units 6-hourly
   b. Increase oxygenation
   c. Shave both groins so that both may be explored if necessary
3. If the diagnosis is in any doubt, then perform an **immediate** arteriogram

Pre-incision
1. Anaesthetic
   a. If fit for general anaesthetic (GA), then GA with endotracheal intubation
   b. If not fit for GA – local anaesthetic (LA) infiltration of the groin with light sedation and analgesia
2. Skin preparation of both groins, abdomen and thighs, exposing both groins
3. Incision
   Longitudinally over site of common femoral artery midway between symphysis pubis and anterior superior iliac spine

Procedure (Fig. 25)
1. Expose common, superficial and profunda femoral arteries
2. Assess the presence of a pulse (if the embolus is lying at the bifurcation of common femoral, then a pulse is palpable proximally but not distally)
3. Place silastic slings around vessels to control blood flow (clamps tend to break up and embolise thrombus and embolus)
4. Perform arteriotomy at femoral bifurcation – remove blood clot/embolus and send for histological examination
5. Fogarty catheter
   a. Initially proximally with a large catheter to establish flow (always check balloon prior to use), then clamp
   b. Then distally down both main vessels to establish back flow with a smaller catheter, then clamp
6. Beware, overinflation of Fogarty catheter balloon can damage vessel intima

Closure
1. Arteriotomy with 4/0 Prolene with a vein patch if the artery is narrow
2. Check distal pulses once the arteriotomy is released
3. Haemostasis
4. Close in layers
5. If embolectomy is delayed then consider fasciotomy

Postoperative management
1. Palpate foot pulses regularly and measure pedal pressures by Doppler
2. Continue to heparinise and subsequently warfarinise
3. Investigate
   a. Histology of embolus (exclude left atrial myxoma)
   b. Echocardiogram to exclude mural thrombus as source of embolism
   c. If echocardiogram negative then aortogram with lateral views

Complications
1. Prognosis if treated within 12 hours, 80% successful
2. If treated later than 12 hours, 20% successful
3. Recurrent thrombosis, especially if acute ischaemia was due to thrombosis on ulcerated atheroma rather than embolism
4. Lymphatic groin fistula/leakage
5. Compartment syndrome if embolectomy delayed

SADDLE EMBOLUS

The same approach is adopted, the exception being that bilateral femoral control is necessary. It is usually possible to remove the embolus intact from one groin with a Fogarty catheter. Access to the other femoral artery is useful if embolectomy on the first side fails and also if the procedure produces subsequent embolism down the other side

Orthopaedic surgery

PRINCIPLES OF SURGERY FOR RHEUMATOID ARTHRITIS

Types of surgery
1. Early rheumatoid synovectomy
   a. Large joints
   b. Metacarpophalangeal joints
2. Intermediate rheumatoid
   a. Divide synovial adhesions
   b. Repair tendons
3. Advanced rheumatoid
   a. Arthrodesis
   b. Arthroplasty
      • Excision
      • Hemi
      • Surface
      • Total

Preoperative management
1. If on steroids, then increase for the duration of the operation and immediate postoperative period
2. Broad spectrum antibiotic cover
3. Beware rheumatoid involving cervical spine resulting in instability. Therefore
   a. Cervical spine X-rays
   b. Support the neck with a cervical collar during the anaesthetic
   c. Consider fixation of the cervical spine

Principles of surgery
1. The aim of surgery is to reduce pain and restore joint function
2. Use straight incisions
3. Delicate tissues must be handled carefully

SPECIFIC SITES

Shoulder
1. Avoid arthrodesis (since further incapacitates the polyarthritic and the bone is often softened)

2. Consider
   a. Synovectomy
   b. Total shoulder replacement (Kessel or Stanmore)

Elbow
1. Synovectomy
2. Excision arthroplasty of the head of the radius
3. Ulnar nerve decompression and transposition (*see* p. 184)
4. Excise rheumatoid nodules
5. Total joint replacement if pain very severe

Hand
1. Carpal tunnel – release (*see* p. 186)
2. Trigger finger – release (excise synovium)
3. Rupture
   a. Repair or reimplant insertion
   b. Tendon transfer (e.g. extensor indicis to extensor pollicis longus)

Tendons
1. Tenosynovitis
2. Tenolysis

Joints
1. MCP
   a. Early – synovectomy
   b. Late – arthroplasty
        – excise MC heads
        – total: Swanson silastic
2. Thereby correcting
   a. Ulnar drift
   b. Dropped heads
3. PIP
   Synovectomy
   a. Reduces pain and swelling
   b. Does not improve function
4. Boutonniere deformity
   a. Early – operate
   b. Late – leave
5. Swan neck deformity
   a. Arthrodesis
   b. Swanson arthroplasty } Equal result
6. DIP – leave

Thumb
1. Ulnar collateral ligament laxity – arthroplasty
2. Carpo metacarpal joint
   a. Arthrodesis
   b. Trapezium replacement (Swanson silastic) equally effective

3. Beware carpal silastic implant dislocation
4. Therefore, plaster of Paris for 6 weeks

Hip
Total hip replacement (*see* p. 192)

Knee
1. Early
    a. Synovectomy
    b. Excise popliteal cyst
2. Late
    a. Arthroplasty
        • Surface
        • Hinge
        • Semi-constrained
    b. Avoid arthrodesis in softened bone
    c. Causes undue stress on other joints

PUTTI PLATT OPERATION FOR RECURRENT DISLOCATION OF THE SHOULDER

Preoperative management
1. Confirm diagnosis by apprehension test – abduction with external rotation
2. Mark the side
3. Check the axillary nerve is intact
4. Investigations – X-rays
    a. AP and lateral in abduction
    b. Arthrogram

Pre-incision
1. General anaesthetic with endotracheal intubation
2. Position – supine
3. Skin preparation of neck to lower chest, axilla, shoulder, arm to elbow
4. Towel up arm separately with shoulder exposed

Incision
Medial border of anterior deltoid to clavicle, then posteriorly to acromion

Procedure
1. Access to joint
    a. Reflect skin flap laterally and retract medially or divide cephalic vein
    b. Explore the delto-pectoral cleft
    c. Divide acromial branch of acromio-thoracic artery between ligatures

    d. Divide proximal deltoid 1 cm from its origin medial to lateral
       for the width of the incision
    e. Retract medially
       • Coracobrachialis
       • Short head of biceps thereby exposing subscapularis and
         its tendon, which is divided 1 cm from its insertion
2. Once the joint is opened, inspect
    a. Inside of the capsule
    b. Head of humerus
    c. Glenoid
    d. Place the arm in 15° of flexion and 90° of internal rotation,
       suture the lateral cuff of subscapularis to the anterior aspect
       of the glenoid with interrupted non-absorbable sutures

Closure
1. Suture medial subscapularis to its lateral tendon superficially
2. Drain – suction deep to deltoid
3. Repair deltoid
4. Skin

Postoperative care
1. Keep arm in internal rotation with a sling to support the elbow
   for 6 weeks
2. Use hand immediately
3. Check position with X-ray

ULNAR NERVE TRANSPOSITION

Indications – ulnar nerve symptoms
1. Following fracture of either condyle of the humerus
2. Osteoarthritis resulting in osteophytes at the elbow
3. Recurrent dislocation of the nerve
4. Excessive carrying angle
5. Idiopathic

Preoperative management
1. Examine, mark the side and fully document any neurological
   deficit (sensory deficit in little, ring finger; weakness of interossi
   with adduction/abduction of fingers)
2. Investigations
    a. PA and lateral X-rays of elbow
    b. EMG studies of ulnar nerve
    c. Sickle test prior to tourniquet in Negroes

Pre-incision
1. General anaesthetic
2. Exsanguinate the arm and apply an arm tourniquet at
   250 mmHg, note the time

3. Position – supine with the arm extended and abducted on a side table
4. Skin preparation of upper arm to wrist

Incision (Fig. 29)
10 cm incision following the ulnar nerve and centred on the medial epicondyle

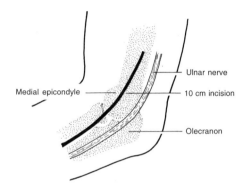

Medial epicondyle

Ulnar nerve

10 cm incision

Olecranon

Fig. 29 Incision for ulnar nerve transposition.

Procedure
1. Expose and mobilise the nerve, carefully preserving its blood supply
2. Incise flexor carpi ulnaris between its two heads. Divide the medial intermuscular septum to expose the nerve
3. Beware: motor branch to flexor carpi ulnaris
4. Separate the common flexor origin from the medial epicondyle and place the nerve anterior to the medial epicondyle

Closure
1. Secure the nerve with interrupted absorbable sutures in the overlying soft tissues
2. Suction drain to the wound
3. Close the skin and apply a firm dressing
4. Release the tourniquet, documenting the tourniquet time

Postoperative management
Encourage early mobilisation

Complications
1. Ulnar nerve neuropraxia should recover quickly
2. Damage motor branch to flexor carpi ulnaris

CARPAL TUNNEL OPERATION

Preoperative management
1. Examine the patient and mark the side, note any neurological deficit, especially to muscles of the thenar eminence
2. Investigations
   a. Exclude aetiological factors – rheumatoid; diabetes
   b. Diagnostic – EMG studies of median nerve function
   c. Sickle status in non-whites prior to tourniquet

Pre-incision
1. General anaesthetic with exsanguination of the arm or Biers block
2. Exsanguinate the arm and inflate an arm tourniquet to 250 mmHg
3. Note the time
4. Position – supine with arm extended on a side table
5. Skin preparation of all of hand and forearm, towel up with hand exposed and extended (assisted by a 'lead hand')

Incision (Fig. 30)
Commencing at distal flexor crease of wrist and extending for 6 cm, 1 cm medial to thenar crease

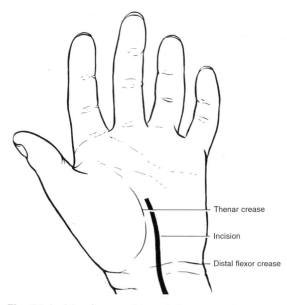

Thenar crease

Incision

Distal flexor crease

Fig. 30 Incision for carpal tunnel decompression.

Procedure
1. Deepen through deep forearm fascia proximally and palmar fascia distally
2. In this medial position the incision should avoid
   a. Proximally – superficial branch of median nerve
   b. Distally – recurrent motor branch of medial nerve to the thenar eminence
3. Visualise the median nerve proximal to the flexor retinaculum lying on the tendons of flexor digitorum sublimis
4. Insert a Macdonald dissector under the proximal border of the flexor retinaculum to protect the median nerve and divide the retinacular fibres longitudinally with a scalpel
5. Direct the division to the ulnar side at its distal end to avoid the recurrent motor branch of the nerve. Divide all the fibres of the retinaculum
6. Gently retract the nerve and flexor tendons to inspect the underlying flexor surface of the carpus for ganglia which should be excised

Closure
1. Close the skin and apply a pressure dressing
2. Release the tourniquet and document the tourniquet time

Postoperative management
1. Can be done as a day case surgery
2. Encourage early activity and keep elevated

Complications
Division of
1. Superficial cutaneous branch of median nerve
2. Recurrent motor branch of median nerve to thenar eminence

EXCISION OF DUPUYTREN'S CONTRACTURE

Indications
Incapacitating Dupuytren's contracture

Preoperative management
Examine and mark the side

Pre-incision
1. General anaesthetic
2. Position – supine with arm extended on a side table
3. Exsanguinate the arm with and inflate an arm tourniquet to a pressure of 250 mmHg, note the time
4. Skin preparation of all of hand and forearm

Incision
1. Mark out a zig-zag incision commencing proximal to the contracture on the palm and extending distal to the contracture on the finger
2. Incise the skin and dissect off the contracture beneath the incision until normal palmar fascia is reached

Procedure
1. Commencing proximally, dissect the abnormal palmar fascia off the deeper structures and continue distally into the finger
2. Divide any adhesions to the fibrous flexor sheath
3. Beware damage to the palmar digital neurovascular bundles

Closure
1. Only drain if dissection is extensive
2. Close the skin loosely
3. Large, firm padded bandage

Postoperative management
Keep elevated for several days and encourage early activity

Complications
Operative
1. Severe finger flexion contracture, either excise the volar capsule or if severely incapacitating obtain consent for amputation
2. Damage to neurovascular bundle

TREATMENT OF HAND INFECTIONS
Superficial
1. 95%
2. Paronychia
3. Subcutaneous abscess
4. Pulp space infection (whitlow)
5. Web space
6. Middle volar infection (may spread and become deep)

Treatment
1. Direct incision to drain pus which should be sent for microbiological examination
2. Appropriate antibiotics for a full therapeutic course
3. Keep hand elevated

Deep
1. 5%
2. Clinically
   a. Swollen throbbing painful hand
   b. Systemically unwell
   c. Greatly diminished movement in hand

3. Suppurating tenosynovitis
   a. Single sheath
   b. Ulnar bursa
   c. Radial bursa
   d. Full therapeutic course of flucloxacillin
   e. Drain synovial sheath both proximally and distally and irrigate the sheath with antibiotic solution
   f. Elevate and encourage early mobilisation to reduce fibrous adhesions within the sheath
4. Fascial space infection
   a. Lateral (thenar) space – incise 1st web posteriorly
   b. Medial (palmar) space – incise directly
   c. Hypothenar space – incise directly
   d. All incisions in skin creases
   e. Divide tissues longitudinally thereby avoiding neurovascular bundles, tendons, etc.
   f. Trim skin edges
   g. Elevate and encourage early mobilisation
5. Complications
   a. Infection
      • Septicaemia
      • Lymphangitis
      • Spread via space of Parona to forearm
   b. Suppurative arthritis
      • Median nerve compression
      • Stiff fingers
   c. Persistent suppuration
      • Foreign body
      • Other sheath/space involved Osteomyelitis
      • Sloughed tendon

LUMBAR LAMINECTOMY

Indications
1. Immediate
   a. Acute central disc protrusion
   b. Acute lateral disc protrusion with lower motor neurone paralysis/sensory deficit
2. Urgent
   a. Acute lateral disc protrusion
   b. Extradural or intradural spinal tumour
   c. Extradural abscess of the spine
3. After conservative management
   a. Chronic disc protrusion
   b. Lumbar spinal stenosis

Preoperative management
1. Full, documented neurological examination
2. Investigations
   a. Plain X-rays – AP and lateral of all of the spine
   b. Myelography
   c. MRI
3. IVI
4. Broad spectrum antibiotics prophylaxis

Pre-incision
1. General anaesthesia with endotracheal intubation
2. Position – prone, with chest and pelvis supported and lumbar spine flexed
3. Skin preparation of all of back, towelled up to expose and midline over the lumbar spine

Incision
Longitudinal 12 cm mid-line centred on the affected disc space

Procedure
1. Deepen the incision to the spinous processes and clean the erector spinae muscles off the spinous processes and laminae on the side of the lesion with cutting diathermy
2. Insert a self-retaining retractor
3. Identify the sacrum which moves with the pelvis and then the lamina overlying the compressed root by counting up from L5/S1 above the sacrum
4. Excise the lower half of the lamina above with bone nibblers
5. Pick up and excise the ligamentum flavum, bounded by the bony margins
6. Identify and retract the dura medially to expose the prolapsed disc
7. Extract the prolapsed disc and curette the disc space
8. Ensure the nerve root now lies free in its foramen

Closure
1. No drains
2. Close
   a. Lumbar fascia
   b. Skin

Postoperative management
Encourage early mobilisation with adequate analgesia

Investigations
1. If for abscess
   Pus for microscopy, culture and sensitivity
2. If for tumour
   Histological examination

Complications

1. Early
   a. Ileus
   b. Acute retention
2. Late
   Recurrent disc if curettage is inadequate

APPROACH TO THE HIP JOINT

Preoperation

1. Examine and mark side
2. Investigations
   a. X-ray of hip
      • AP
      • Lateral
3. Broad spectrum antibiotic prophylaxis

Pre-incision

General anaesthesia with endotracheal intubation

POSTERIOR APPROACH (Fig. 31)

1. Position – lateral with pillow between legs
2. Skin preparation loin to knee with U drape in groin and leg towelled separately

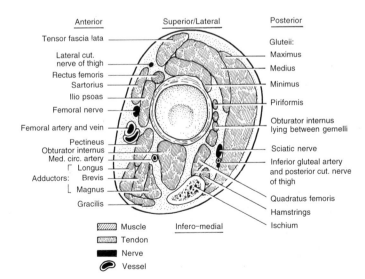

Fig. 31 Anatomical relations of hip joint.

Incision
20 cm long centred on greater trochanter curved superiorly towards posterior superior iliac spine

Procedure
1. Deepen incision including fascia/ilio tibial tract
2. Divide insertion of gluteus maximus to posterior aspect of greater trochanter separating anterior border to gluteus maximus from gluteus medius
3. Divide insertions of
   a. Obturator internus with gemelli
   b. Quadratus femoris and reflect posteriorly – thereby protecting the sciatic nerve lying posteriorly
4. Beware sciatic nerve posteriorly
5. Perform capsulotomy
6. Incise the exposed capsule and dislocate hip with internal rotation and flexion with adduction

ANTERIOR APPROACH
1. Position – supine
2. Skin preparation of loin to knee, U drape to perineum and towel up with leg free

Incision
Anterior superior iliac spine to greater trochanter and continue laterally 10 cm along thigh

Procedure
1. Deepen incision to fascia lata/ilio tibial tract
2. Deepen between sartorius and tensor fascia lata, dividing origin of sartorius
3. Beware lateral circumflex iliac vessels
4. Divide origin of rectus femoris near anterior superior iliac spine to display capsule
5. Perform capsulotomy
6. Dislocate hip with external rotation

Closure
1. Drain
   a. To joint
   b. To wound
2. Close in layers

TOTAL HIP REPLACEMENT
Indications
1. Osteoarthritis
2. Rheumatoid arthritis

Preoperative management
1. Exclude sites of chronic sepsis
2. Examine and mark the side
3. Broad spectrum antibiotic prophylaxis intravenously with induction achieves best bone levels
4. IVI
5. Catheterise if appropriate

Pre-incision
As for approach to the hip (*see* p. 191), either approach is acceptable

Procedure
1. Perform capsulotomy and dislocate the joint
2. Excise the joint capsule
3. Divide the femoral neck in a line obliquely 1–2 cm above the greater trochanter. Cut the ligamentum teres to remove the head
4. Ream the acetabulum down to bone until it is large enough to accept the acetabular prosthesis
5. Drill two or three keyholes in the acetabulum (one into each of the ilium, ischium and pubis)
6. Prepare the methyl methacrylate bone cement and fix the acetabular component
7. Prepare further bone cement and fix the femoral component
8. Reduce the hip

Closure
As for approach to the hip (*see* p. 191)

Postoperative management
1. Investigation
   Check X-rays of reduction
2. Mobilise after 2 days

Complications
1. Operative
   a. Fracture of femoral shaft
   b. Penetration of acetabulum into pelvis
   c. Wrong acetabular geometry allowing post-reduction dislocation
   d. Hypotension with implantation of cement
2. Postoperative
   a. Infection
      • May result in loosening
      • Salvage with Girdlestones operation
   b. Loosening
      • Infection
      • Reduce with high pressure cement injections
   c. Calcification in soft tissues around prosthesis

OPEN MEDIAL MENISCECTOMY

Preoperative preparation
1. Examine and mark the side
2. Commence quadriceps exercises
3. Negro needs Sickle test for tourniquet
4. X-rays/arthrograms of knee
5. Arthroscopy

Pre-incision
1. General anaesthetic with endotracheal intubation. Exsanguinate leg and apply a tourniquet to affected thigh at 500 mmHg pressure and note time
2. Position
   Supine with legs unsupported below the flexed knees
3. Skin preparation of upper thigh to ankle with lower leg towelled separately and knee draped in op-site or sterile tubular bandage
4. Surgeon
   Seated facing affected knee with the foot in his lap

Incision
Vertical, medial to patella and its tendon from above knee to level with tibial tubercle

Procedure
1. Incise capsule in the line of the incision and retract medially
2. Assess
   a. Medial meniscus
   b. Joint – loose bodies
   c. Osteochondritis
   d. Arthritic changes
3. Divide anterior horn, grasping meniscus with Kocher's forceps
4. Divide capsular attachment with a Smillie knife
5. Detach posterior horn by sharp dissection

Postoperative management
1. Encourage early mobilisation, non weight bearing
2. Ordinary shoes can be worn after about 3 months

Complications
1. Hallux dorsiflexion deformity
   Needs lengthening plastic procedure of extensor hallucis longus
2. Persistent valgus deformity
   Fix the truncated proximal phalanx to the metatarsal head with a longitudinal Kirschner wire to encourage fibrous ankylosis in that position

ZADEK'S OPERATION

Indications
Chronic ingrowing great toe nail

Contraindications
1. Sepsis
2. Peripheral vascular disease

Preoperative management
1. Examine and mark the side
2. Exclude diabetes as a contributory factor in recurrent infection

Pre-incision
1. Either general or local ring block (*avoid adrenaline*) anaesthesia
2. Position – supine
3. Skin preparation of all of foot, apply a rubber tourniquet to the proximal hallux

Procedure
1. Remove the toe nail
2. Make two oblique incisions into the skin at each corner of the nail bed for 0.5–1 cm
3. Retract the skin off the germinal matrix of the nail root for the whole of its width
4. Excise the nail matrix underlying the skin for its whole width down to periosteum
5. Beware leaving pockets of nail matrix in each corner

Closure
1. Suture the two skin incisions
2. Dress the wound with a non-adherent dressing
3. Release the tourniquet and check re-establishment of the circulation

Postoperative management
This can be done as day case surgery

Complications
Recurrent ingrowth of spikes of nail left from residual germinal matrix in the corners

SITES OF MAJOR JOINT ASPIRATION

Wrist
Posteriorly, between extensor pollicis longus and extensor indicis

Elbow
1. Postero laterally
   Above radial head
2. Posteriorly
   In mid-line

Shoulder
Anteriorly by medial border of deltoid (avoid cephalic vein)

Hip
1. Anteriorly
   2.5 cm below and lateral to mid-inguinal point (beware femoral artery and nerve)
2. Laterally
   Just above the tip of the greater trochanter, then pass upwards and medially over the femoral neck

Knee
Either medial or lateral to patellar tendon

Ankle
Anterior to lateral malleolus

Investigations
1. If for abscess
   Pus for microscopy, culture and sensitivity
2. If for gout
   Microscopy for crystals

Trauma surgery

LAPAROTOMY FOR ABDOMINAL TRAUMA

Resuscitate

1. Airway
2. Breathing
3. Circulation – peripheral IVIs
   a. At least two large bore cannulae
   b. Cross-match at least 6 units of blood urgently
   c. Commence crystalloid infusion if stable or colloid infusion if haemodynamically unstable

Assess

1. Catheterise
   Haematuria – proceed to IVP with continuous Conray infusion (*see* Principles of urological trauma management, p. 206)
2. Rectal examination
3. Plain abdominal X-rays
   a. Foreign bodies
   b. Free gas
4. Beware effects of cavitation shock waves transmitted by the great vessels following high velocity missile injuries to limbs
5. Peritoneal lavage is approximately 90% accurate in detecting significant intraperitoneal haemorrhage (false positive rate 2–3%)
   a. Infiltrate 10–20 cc 1% lignocaine into the abdominal mid-line below the umbilicus
   b. Make a 4–5 cm mid-line incision down to the linea alba
   c. Incise the linea alba for 2–3 cm to expose the preperitoneal fat
   d. Expose the peritoneum and place the peritoneal dialysis catheter into the peritoneum *under direct vision*
   e. Run in up to 500 cc of normal saline and then place infusion bag on the floor to syphon back the peritoneal lavage solution
   f. If uniformly blood stained then suspect significant intraperitoneal bleeding and proceed to laparotomy

6. Careful repeated observations
7. A patient who is haemodynamically unstable following blunt abdominal trauma should proceed as soon as is physically possible to laparotomy

Indications for laparotomy
1. All penetrating wounds (no matter how superficial they appear in the casualty department)
2. Blunt abdominal trauma
   a. Hypovolaemic shock
   b. Free gas on plain abdominal X-rays
   c. Clothing imprintation on the skin
   d. Peritonism
   e. Blood stained peritoneal lavage
3. Beware concomitant major injury
   a. Pelvic fracture
   b. Chest (*see* Management of major chest trauma, p. 201)
      • Flail segment
      • Adult respiratory distress syndrome
      • Intrapleural tension
   c. Head (*see* p. 212)

Pre-procedure
1. In profound hypovolaemia, do not delay surgery in an attempt to restore the blood pressure
2. Broad spectrum and metronidazole antibiotic cover
3. Antitetanus measures

Pre-incision
1. General anaesthesia and endotracheal intubation, induced once the patient is on the operating table
   a. Central venous pressure monitor } Can wait until surgery
   b. Arterial line   is under way
2. Position
   a. Supine
   b. Upper abdominal trauma – consider thoracoabdominal approach
3. Skin preparation of all of abdomen from above the nipples to mid thigh

Incision
Excise and close penetrating wound, then proceed to laparotomy

Procedure
1. Needs full laparotomy
2. Profuse bleeding
   a. Evacuate clots

   b. Systematically pack off all four quadrants with large
      abdominal swabs and then remove to localise the source of
      the bleeding
3. Kocherise the duodenum
   a. Posterior duodenum
   b. Posterior head of pancreas
   c. IVC
   d. Right renal area
4. Open both lateral colic peritoneal reflections to examine the
   posterior ascending and descending colon
5. Examine the pelvis
   a. Urological trauma (*see* p. 206)
   b. Rectal injury
      • Drain pelvis
      • Proximal colostomy
      • Drain presacral area externally by excising coccyx

INJURY TO SPECIFIC ORGANS

Small bowel and mesentery (Fig. 32)

1. Perforation
   a. Small – repair
   b. Large – resect
2. Mesenteric tear

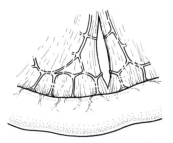

Longitudinal mesenteric tear - repair

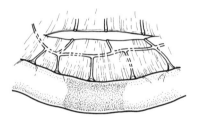

Transverse mesenteric tear resulting in devitalisation - resect

Fig. 32 Longitudinal
and transverse
mesenteric tears.

a. Transverse – resect as vessels often involved
b. Longitudinal – repair

Large bowel
1. Avoid primary resection with anastomosis
2. Caecum
   a. Right hemicolectomy with ileostomy and mucous fistula
   b. Transverse/descending colon – excise with proximal colostomy and mucous fistula

Liver
1. Profuse bleeding
   Pringle's manoeuvre (pinch hepatic artery and portal vein in right free border of lesser omentum)
2. *See* Hepatic resection (p. 101)

Spleen
1. Small tear – consider repair and preservation
2. Large tear – splenectomy (*see* p. 94)

Retroperitoneum
1. Duodenum
   a. Kocherise and examine fully
   b. Repair and drain perforation
2. Pancreas
   a. Head
      • Small – drain
      • Large – consider resection
   b. Tail
      • Small – drain
      • Large – resect with spleen
3. Haematoma
   a. Small – leave
   b. Large – evacuate and drain
4. Kidney (*see* Urological trauma, p. 206)

Problems
1. Severe uncontrollable pelvic bleeding – consider angiography and embolisation of pelvic vessels
2. Severe liver injury
   a. May need right thoracotomy to control caval bleeding
   b. Transfer to regional hepatobiliary unit

Multiple injuries
10% have abdominal injuries – 25% mortality
    a. Of these
        • 10–30% have thoracic injuries – 40% mortality
        • 30% have pelvic injuries – 30% mortality
        • 30% have leg injuries – 30% mortality
        • 20% have head injuries – 50% mortality
    b. Major abdominal, chest and head injury – 80% mortality
(Consider tracheostomy (*see* p. 34)

Postoperative management
1. Once stable, transfer to regional trauma/specialist unit if necessary
2. Nurse on an intensive care unit
3. Monitor
    a. Pulse
    b. Blood pressure
    c. CVP ± pulmonary artery wedge pressure
    d. Urine output
    e. Packed cell volume/haemoglobin and transfuse accordingly

Complications
1. Acute renal failure
2. Adult respiratory distress syndrome
3. Infection
    a. Peritonitis
    b. Wound
    c. Abscess
    d. Septicaemia
    e. Respiratory tract
    f. *Clostridia*
4. Disseminated intravascular coagulation
5. Upper gastrointestinal bleeding

MANAGEMENT OF MAJOR CHEST TRAUMA
Resuscitate
(*See* Abdominal trauma, p. 197)
1. Airway
2. Breathing
3. Circulation
    a. At least two IVIs
    b. Cross match 10 units of blood
4. Drain to relieve tension
    a. Pleura
    b. Pericardium
5. Excise and close wounds

Management

1. 90% of blunt chest trauma can be managed conservatively
2. 80% of penetrating chest wounds can be managed by excision and primary wound closure with underwater seal drainage if penetrating beyond parietal pleura

Problems

1. Penetrating wounds frequently do not occur in isolation
2. Chest and neck
   a. Brachial plexus
   b. Carotid sheath structures
   c. Thoracic duct on left
   d. Trachea/oesophagus
3. Chest and abdomen
   Needs thoracoabdominal exposure (*see* Laparotomy for abdominal trauma, p. 197)
4. Blunt injuries
   a. Concomitant spinal and pelvic injury
   b. Head injury (*see* Craniotomy for extradural haematoma, p. 212)
   c. Abdominal injury (*see* Laparotomy for abdominal trauma, p. 197)

Specific intrathoracic problems

1. Great vessels, especially with crushing chest injury (*see* Vascular trauma management, p. 203)
2. Chest wall: flail/stove in injury, manage with intubation and positive pressure ventilation
3. Pleura
   a. Pneumothorax
      • Simple
      • Tension
   b. Haemothorax
      • Usually from intercostal vessels
4. Pericardial tamponade
5. Direct myocardial damage – needs 12-lead ECG
6. Trachea/main bronchus fracture – repair

Exploration

1. Use posterolateral thoracotomy (*see* p. 51)
2. Never use positive pressure ventilation until pleural drains are in place, when there is a suspicion of pneumothorax

3. Indications for thoracotomy
   a. Excessive uncontrollable bleeding
   b. Excessive air leak from broncho-pleural
      fistula
   c. Penetrating wound to mediastinum/pericardium
   d. Tamponade
   e. Thoracoabdominal injury
   f. Chest wall defect
4. Relative indications for thoracotomy sucking chest
   wall wound
5. Antibiotic cover
   a. Broad spectrum and flucloxacillin
   b. Tetanus cover
6. Consider transfer to regional cardiothoracic centre
   once stable

VASCULAR TRAUMA MANAGEMENT

Assessment
1. Always suspect
   a. All limb injuries especially fractures of long
      bones
   b. Enlarging/pulsating haematoma
   c. Distal vascular insufficiency (diminished pulse or Doppler
      pressure)
2. Manage life threatening problems before limb threatening
   problems
3. Venous injury is as important as arterial injury
4. Clinical examination of arteries
   a. Pulses present?
   b. Pulse pressure
      • Auscultation
      • Doppler
   c. Evidence of ischaemic cutaneous anaesthesia
5. Presence of Doppler arterial pulse does not exclude arterial
   disruption
6. X-rays
   a. Plain in two planes at 90° to each other
      • Fracture
      • Foreign body
   b. Arteriogram when there *is any doubt* about the presence of,
      or site of, arterial injury
7. *Never ascribe arterial disruption to*
   spasm

Principles of management
1. Control haemorrhage with direct pressure
2. Prevent infection
   a. Antisepsis, debridement, antitetanus
   b. Broad spectrum antibiotic with flucloxacillin
3. Stabilise fracture
   Consider indwelling shunt in artery if delay in reconstruction likely
4. Restore circulation
   a. General anaesthetic
   b. Good exposure of injury
   c. Good control of arteries and veins both proximally and distally
   d. Evacuate haematoma
5. Repair
   Options
   a. End-to-end anastomosis of divided vessels; suture of incised injury
   b. Vein patch over defect
   c. Extensive defect – insert reverse vein graft (vein from uninjured limb)
6. Local anticoagulation with heparin in saline (5000 units in 500 cc normal saline)
7. Reassess veins after restoring arterial supply
   a. Debride wound
   b. Cover arterial repair
   c. Do not close contaminated wounds

Indications for fasciotomy
1. Extensive soft tissue damage
2. Swelling
3. >6 hours delay after injury/embolism
4. Combined arteriovenous injury
5. Any popliteal vessel trauma procedure
   a. Decompress all compartments (in the leg this can be achieved by fibula excision)
   b. Volkmanns type of ischaemia will occur with a tissue hydrostatic pressure of >50 mmHg, and therefore can arise in the presence of palpable peripheral pulses
   c. Postoperatively
   Needs regular review of ischaemic limb, re-explore if any evidence of diminishing circulation

SPECIFIC ARTERIAL PROBLEMS

Thoracic aorta
1. Deceleration injuries (car driver)
2. Usually between left subclavian artery and ligamentum arteriosum
3. 20% will survive to reach hospital and may have good equal femoral pulses
4. Investigations
   a. Diagnosis on suspicion from the history
   b. CXR
      • Widening aorta
      • Depressed left main bronchus
      • NG tube displaced to right
   c. Arch aortogram
5. Preoperative neurological examination of legs
6. Proceed to surgery in a cardiac unit if possible, therefore cardiopulmonary bypass feasible
7. Simple bypass is possible with a silastic catheter between the apex of the left ventricle and descending aorta
8. Beware associated injuries
   a. Myocardial contusion
   b. Adult respiratory distress syndrome
   c. Multiple injuries
   d. Paraplegia due to spinal cord ischaemia

Femoral artery
1. Often occurs in association with venous injury
2. Common femoral – rare
   a. Penetrating – butcher's knife
   b. Orthopaedic procedure
3. Superficial femoral
   a. Common – fractured femur
   b. Treatment
      • Ligation – 50% amputation rate
      • Repair – 10% amputation rate

Popliteal artery
60% have associated popliteal vein injury
1. Associated with
   a. Direct trauma
   b. Knee dislocation
   c. Menisectomy
2. Repair artery and reconstruct veins
   <20% amputation
3. Ligate artery
   80% amputation rate
4. *Always requires full length, four compartment fasciotomy*

Brachial artery
Common iatrogenic injury (following cardiac
catheterisation)
1. Associated nerve injury
   a. Ischaemic
   b. Direct trauma to median and ulnar nerve
2. Always reconstruct

PRINCIPLES OF UROLOGICAL TRAUMA MANAGEMENT
RENAL TRAUMA
Establish diagnosis
1. History
   a. Blunt trauma
   b. Penetrating injury
2. Examination
   a. Bruising/laceration
   b. Haematoma
   c. Haematuria
3. Associated injury
   a. Fractured ribs
   b. Spleen/liver (*see* Splenectomy, p. 94 and Principles of hepatic
      resection, p. 101) and lung (*see* Management of major chest
      trauma, p. 201)
   c. Spine
4. Abdominal X-ray
   a. Loss or renal/psoas shadow
   b. Fractured lower ribs
   c. Protective scoliosis
   d. Soft tissue mass (haematoma)

Antibiotics
Broad spectrum

IVU
By continuous Conray infusion

Management

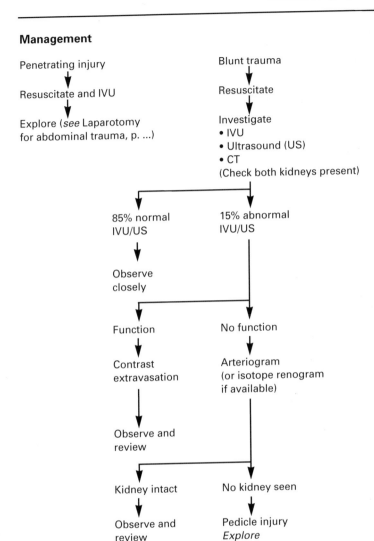

Penetrating injury

Resuscitate and IVU

Explore (*see* Laparotomy
for abdominal trauma, p. ...)

Blunt trauma

Resuscitate

Investigate
- IVU
- Ultrasound (US)
- CT
(Check both kidneys present)

85% normal
IVU/US

Observe
closely

15% abnormal
IVU/US

Function

Contrast
extravasation

No function

Arteriogram
(or isotope renogram
if available)

Observe and
review

Kidney intact

Observe and
review

No kidney seen

Pedicle injury
Explore

80% have damage to other viscera

Renal injury
Drain renal bed and nephrostomy to protect kidney from clot bolus
obstruction of ureter

If the pedicle is completely severed, consider autotransplant unless
the kidney is totally disrupted, then remove

BLADDER TRAUMA

Establish diagnosis
1. Blunt trauma
   a. Direct blow to full bladder usually causes intraperitoneal rupture
   b. Fractured pelvis (beware associated urethural injury) may cause extraperitoneal rupture
2. Penetrating injury
   a. Stab wound
   b. Iatrogenic
      - Endoscopic surgery
      - Pelvic surgery
      - Hernia repair (especially strangulated)

Presents with anuria/scanty blood stained urine

Investigations
1. AXR
   a. Fractured pelvis
   b. Ground glass appearance with intraperitoneal perforation
2. IVU
   a. May show extravasation of contrast
   b. Cystography if no urethral injury

Management
Resuscitate
If no obvious urethral injury - catheterise

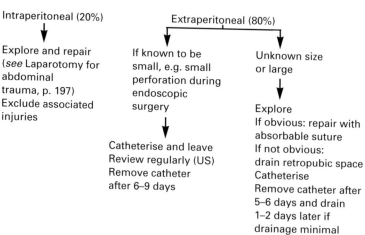

Intraperitoneal (20%)

Explore and repair
(*see* Laparotomy for
abdominal
trauma, p. 197)
Exclude associated
injuries

Extraperitoneal (80%)

If known to be
small, e.g. small
perforation during
endoscopic
surgery

Catheterise and leave
Review regularly (US)
Remove catheter
after 6–9 days

Unknown size
or large

Explore
If obvious: repair with
absorbable suture
If not obvious:
drain retropubic space
Catheterise
Remove catheter after
5–6 days and drain
1–2 days later if
drainage minimal

MALE URETHRAL INJURIES

Establish diagnosis
1. History of either fall astride injury (bulbar urethra) or pelvic injury (membranous urethra) with inability to pass urine (beware neurogenic acute retention with concomitant spinal injury)
2. Inability to pass urine after traumatic endoscopic surgery
3. Blood at external meatus ± perineal bruising
4. Beware associated bladder injury

Investigations
1. Plain pelvic X-rays
2. IVU
3. Avoid urethrogram, may convert an incomplete rupture into a complete rupture
4. An experienced urologist may try one attempt to pass a fine, soft urethral catheter into the bladder

Urinary extravasation
1. Prostatic urethral injury
   a. Deep to muscles of anterior abdominal wall and triangular ligament
   b. Within fascia of Denonvilliers
2. Bulbar urethral injury
   a. Deep to Scarpa's fascia
   b. Within Colles' fascia

MANAGEMENT OF MALE URETHRAL INJURIES

History
1. Injury to bulbar urethra below external sphincter (fall astride)
2. Haematoma or urinary extravasation
3. Unable to pass urine

Management
1. Suprapubic catheter if inexperienced urologist
2. Subsequently unable to pass urine; refer to urologist
3. Subsequently passes urine: urethrogram at 3 weeks to exclude stricture
4. Able to pass urine: leave and review
5. Manage subsequent stricture
6. Beware extravasation

Injury to membranous/prostatic urethra above external sphincter (usually with associated pelvic injury)
1. Able to pass urine
   Urethrogram at 3 weeks to exclude stricture
2. Beware urinary extravasation

3. Unable or difficult to pass urine
   Explore
   a. Complete disruption
   b. Floating bladder
      • Repair by Turner Warwick method
      • Manage subsequent stricture
4. Incomplete urethral disruption with bladder in place
   a. Repair bladder
   b. Suprapubic catheter
   c. Drain retropubic space
   d. Manage subsequent stricture

MANAGEMENT OF LIMB TRAUMA

Assess
1. All pulses
2. Nerves
   a. Motor
   b. Sensory
3. Beware missile injuries with only small entry wounds causing cavitation effects and destroying collateral circulation (*see* Laparotomy for abdominal trauma, p. 197)
4. Investigations
   a. Plain X-rays in at least two planes including joint above and joint below
   b. Arteriography if vascular injury suspected (*see* Vascular trauma management, p. 203)
5. Full antimicrobial prophylaxis
   a. Antitetanus measures
   b. Broad spectrum antibiotics and flucloxacillin with penicillin for *clostridia*
   c. Aseptic techniques
   d. Antiseptics with full debridement (*avoid alcohol, may irreparably damage nerves and tendons*)

Procedure
Needs
1. Good regional or general anaesthesia
2. Good exposure – using longitudinal incisions and preserving skin
3. Good light

Vascular injuries
(*See* Vascular trauma management, p. 203)
1. Always reconstruct both arteries and veins
2. Beware high velocity missile injury destroying collateral circulation
3. Always needs full length fasciotomies

Nerves
(*See* Principles of management of nerve and tendon injury, p. 220)
1. Simple laceration – primary repair if possible
2. Otherwise label with nonabsorbable suture and close; attempt delayed primary repair at 6 weeks

Muscle
1. If viability doubtful – excise
2. Prevent
   a. Infection (especially gas gangrene)
   b. Contractures (ischaemia, immobility)

Tendons
(*See* Principles of management of nerve and tendon injury, p. 220)
1. Single
   Consider repair
2. Multiple
   Consider repair, but if not experienced then label with nonabsorbable sutures for delayed repair after skin cover completed

Bone
1. Preserve all fragments, curetting and scraping out any debris
2. Irrigate with antiseptic solution
3. Beware internal fixation with contaminated compound fractures

Joints
1. Exposure needs tourniquet control
2. Remove all debris with debridement
3. Irrigate
4. Always close synovium (substitute muscle or skin if synovium lost)

At end of procedure
1. Liberally apply antiseptic soaked dressings
2. Never close if any risk of contamination or with gunshot wounds
3. Elevate

Traumatic amputation
1. Guillotine – consider reimplantation
2. Avulsion/ragged transection
   a. Needs total debridement
   b. Leave open
      • Allows drainage
      • Protect skin edges
   c. Delayed primary closure

Hand/foot
1. Fully decompress and debride wound
2. Leave open and elevate until all swelling reduced
3. Then close/skin graft as soon as possible

If wound left open
1. Examine under anaesthetic on the fifth day, if clean, consider closure/skin grafts
2. Never close under tension

CRANIOTOMY FOR EXTRADURAL HAEMATOMA

Preoperative management
1. Informed consent from relative
2. Investigations
   a. Skull X-rays
   b. CT scan
   c. Ultrasound
3. Preparation
   Shave head completely
4. Antibiotics
   Benzyl penicillin/sulphonamides
5. IVI (beware fluid overload)
6. Catheterise
7. NG tube (both for aspiration and postoperative feeding)
8. Endotracheal tube, preoperatively PaO_2 and $PaCO_2$ by hyperventilation to reduce intracranial pressure

Pre-incision
1. General anaesthesia with endotracheal intubation
2. Avoid inhalation of anaesthetic gases, especially **halothane** since they increase intracranial pressure
3. Position – supine

Incision (Fig. 33)
1. Preauricular: from zygoma to above temple, deepen through all layers to pericranium
2. Separate fibres of temporalis
3. Avoid facial nerve – especially temporal branch

Procedure
1. Insert self-restraining retractor and visualise fracture in superficial temporal bone
2. Commence burr anterior to fracture line with 16 mm Hudson brace to superficial table and with burr to inner table
3. Extradural haematoma should now be visible
4. Extend burr hole with bone nibblers to beyond edge of haematoma

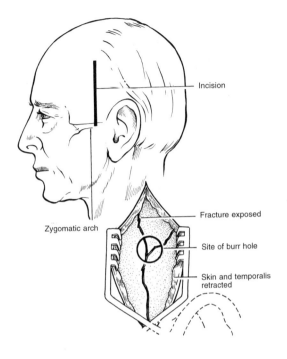

Fig. 33 Craniotomy for extradural haematoma.

5. Remove haematoma from the edge first with sucker (clearing clot from junction of bone and dura)
6. The intracranial pressure should decrease and the clot commence to pulsate as the arterial circulation improves
7. As the clot is removed, the intracranial pressure continues to decrease and the bleeding correspondingly increases
8. Remove centre of clot over bleeding point on middle meningeal artery and ligate with a non-absorbable suture (beware catching the middle cerebral artery lying immediately below the dura with this suture!)

Complications
1. Burr reveals no haematoma but bulging dura – do not open further since results in cerebral herniation
2. Avoid exploratory burrs around cranium and refer for CT scan

Closure
1. Suture dura to temporalis muscle all around edge of craniectomy

2. Haemostasis
3. Close scalp in layers
4. If tracheostomy necessary, best to perform immediately
   (*see* p. 35)

Postoperative management
1. Quarter-hourly neurological observation
2. Ventilate to maintain
   a. High PaO_2
   b. Low $PaCO_2$
3. Tracheostomy/endotracheal tube care
4. Physiotherapy (chest and passive limb movement), intensive nursing care
5. Continue antibiotics for one week
6. Investigation
   If dura opened – daily lumbar puncture for microbiological examination

MANAGEMENT OF FRACTURE NECK OF FEMUR
Preoperative management
1. Examine and mark the side
2. Investigations
   a. Plain X-rays of hip
   b. AP
   c. Lateral
3. Establish the site of fracture (see Fig. 34)
   a. Subcapital
   b. Neck
   c. Trochanteric
4. Catheterise
5. IVI
6. Broad spectrum antibiotic prophylaxis intravenously at induction achieves highest bone levels

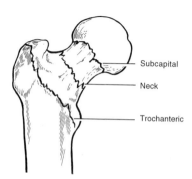

Subcapital

Neck

Trochanteric

Fig. 34 Fractures of neck of femur.

Pre-incision
Either general anaesthesia with endotracheal intubation or
spinal anaesthesia

TROCHANTERIC AND UNDISPLACED SUBCAPITAL (GARDEN I
AND II) FRACTURE OF THE FEMUR
1. Position
    a. Supine on an orthopaedic operating table abducting the
       good leg and reducing the fracture by traction, 10°
       abduction and internal rotation to the affected leg
    b. Set up X-ray image intensifier to be able to view the hip
       in both AP and lateral views
2. Skin preparation from knee to upper abdomen
3. Drape up to allow exposure to lateral upper thigh with
   access for image intensifier (or use Fitzgerald polythene
   'sail')

Incision
20 cm commencing posterior to greater trochanter and
extending longitudinally down the thigh

Procedure
(*See* Approaches to the Hip Joint, p. 191)
   1. Divide fascia lata in the line of the incision
   2. Divide upper origin of vastus lateralis and separate from
      upper lateral femur
   3. Select a site on the lower posterior margin of the greater
      trochanter and cut a small hole in the cortex
   4. Pass two or more guide wires up through the fracture line
      along the posterior inferior part of the femoral neck to lie
      in the femoral head
   5. Beware guide wire penetration of the pelvis
   6. Check the position of the guide wires with the image
      intensifier and select the best positioned. Measure the
      length of guide wire in bone and choose a nail 1 cm
      shorter
   7. Ream the cortex around the insertion of the guide wire
   8. Hammer in the selected nail (e.g. McLaughlin or McKee)
      along the guide wire
   9. Recheck the position of the nail radiologically
  10. Clear the periosteum off the lateral femoral shaft
      for 15 cm
  11. Holding the plate to the femoral shaft, apply the plate to
      the butt of the nail. Secure the plate to the nail with the
      appropriate nut
  12. Secure the plate to the femoral shaft with at least 5 screws
      through both cortices

Closure
1. Suction drain
2. Close in layers

DISPLACED SUBCAPITAL (GARDEN III AND IV) FRACTURED NECK OF FEMUR

Needs hemiarthroplasty

Procedure
1. Needs full exposure of the hip joint (*see* p. 191)
2. Remove head of femur and measure to select suitable size of prosthesis
3. Excise redundant neck of femur at greater trochanter and ream medulla for prosthesis (use either uncemented Austin Moore prosthesis or Thompson's prosthesis with cement)
4. Insert prosthesis dry and perform trial reduction; then if necessary cement prosthesis
5. Reduce hip
6. Test stability
7. Close according to approach (shown on p. 191)

Postoperative management
Encourage early mobilisation

Complications
1. Operative
   a. Nail plate method
      • Penetration of pelvis with nail
      • Damage to profunda femoris with screws to plate
   b. Hemiarthroplasty
      • Fracture of femoral shaft during insertion of prosthesis

Postoperative
1. DVT
2. Bronchopneumonia
3. Dislocation of hemiarthroplasty
4. Loosening of prosthesis

K-NAIL FOR FRACTURED FEMUR

Preoperative
1. Resuscitate
   a. Transfuse to correct hypovolaemia and haemoglobin
   b. Stabilise femur with traction (skin or skeletal with 10 kg)
2. Examine and mark side
3. Measure length of good femur (to choose length of nail) shave thigh and buttock

4. Broad spectrum and flucloxacillin antibiotic prophylaxis
5. IVI

Pre-incision
1. Either spinal or general anaesthesia with endotracheal intubation
2. Position – lateral
3. Surgeon
   Posterior to patient
4. Skin preparation
   a. Mid-abdomen, groin, buttock to below knee
   b. Thigh and buttock exposed
5. Drape to perineum

Incisions
1. Lateral approach to mid-femur 20–30 cm in length
2. Over greater trochanter

Procedure
Mid thigh
1. Deepen between vastus lateralis and intermuscular septum
2. Ligate perforating vessels
3. Assess
   a. Fracture
   b. Soft tissue
   c. Fragments
   d. Reduce, assess stability
4. Beware
   a. Sciatic nerve posteriorly
   b. Excessive traction to leg
5. Ream upper fragments and measure medullary diameter to select width of nail
6. Trochanteric incision
   a. Pass nail over guide wire through greater trochanter into upper fragment as far as fracture
   b. Ream lower fragment to femoral condyles
   c. Reduce fracture
   d. Pass nail the full length of the femur into the lower fragment

Closure
1. Suction drainage to both wounds
2. Close in layers

Postoperative care
1. Investigation X-ray of femur
   a. Reduction
   b. Position of nail

2. Mobilise gently
   a. Practise straight leg raising, walking, non-weight-bearing with crutches at 1–2 weeks
   b. Weight-bearing 4–6 weeks
   c. ?Remove nail at 12–18 months

Complications
1. Infection
   a. Nail
   b. Wounds
2. Fracture
   a. Delayed union
   b. Non-union
   c. Mal union
   d. Nail displacement
3. DVT/PE (*see* Principles of prevention of DVT, p. 7)

MANAGEMENT OF FRACTURED SHAFT OF TIBIA

OPEN FRACTURE

1. Avoid primary closure
   a. Debride wound and antisepsis
   b. External fixation
2. Broad spectrum antibiotic cover
3. Antitetanus measure
4. Examine under anaesthetic 5 days later, then close or graft skin if not infected

CLOSED FRACTURE

Methods

Reduce with manipulation under anaesthesia
1. Place in a split plaster of Paris cast from mid thigh to mid tarsus, well padded with orthopaedic gauze
2. Prevent rotation of fracture components
3. Monitor
   a. Swelling and distal circulation
   b. Displacement
   c. Union/consolidation
4. Complication
   a. Compartment syndrome – needs fasciotomy
   b. Delayed/non union
   c. Mal union

Os-calcis traction
1. 4 kg traction via a Denham pin placed through the os calcis
2. Support the leg on a pillow for 2 weeks

3. Monitor
   a. Soft tissues
   b. Skin
   c. Peripheral circulation
   d. After 2 weeks either – internally fixate or cast brace
4. Complications
   Subtalar joint stiffness

External fixation of the fragments
1. Allows
   a. Adjustment/compression of components
   b. Skin grafting
2. Stability results in better soft tissue healing
3. Complication
4. Infection

Indications for internal fixation
1. Other injuries which preclude above alternatives (e.g. femoral fracture)
2. Old age – needs rapid mobilisation
3. Irreducible/unholdable fracture
4. Failure of above methods
5. Social (time in hospital/financial)

INTERNAL FIXATION OF FRACTURED TIBIA

1. Protect leg by placing in skin or skeletal traction
2. Mark the side
3. Investigation
   X-rays of tibia including knee and ankle joint in two planes at right angles
4. Preparation
   Shave the leg
5. Broad spectrum and flucloxacillin antibiotic prophylaxis

Pre-incision
1. General anaesthetic
2. Avoid tourniquet
3. Position – supine
4. Skin preparation of mid-thigh to foot
5. Towel up with skin exposed, foot covered but mobile

Incision
Longitudinal along skin

Procedure
1. Elevate periosteum and display fracture line
2. Clean bone ends with minimal disturbance of callus and remove interposing soft tissues
3. Attempt reduction and brace fragments together

4. Position a template specific to fracture, sufficient to take at least four screws through both cortices in both proximal and distal fragments
5. Adjust plate to the shape of the tibia and apply to bone, tapping screw holes
6. Screw the plate to the fragments with an optional screw through the fracture line if it is oblique

Closure
1. Suction drainage to plate
2. Close in layers
   a. Periosteum over plate
   b. Skin
3. Split POP cylinder (allows early mobilisation)

Postoperative care
Check position of fragments on X-ray in two planes

Complications
1. Early
   a. Skin damage (especially lower third fracture)
   b. Infection
   c. Compartment syndrome (anterior compartment)
   d. Haematoma
2. Late especially with
   a. Fracture
      • Delayed or non-union damaged nutrient artery to lower third
   b. Joint stiffness, if mobilisation delayed

PRINCIPLES OF MANAGEMENT OF NERVE AND TENDON INJURY
All lacerations need accurate assessment

Accurate history
Position of hand at the time of injury since if in flexion with a flexor surface injury the tendons will retract

Management of sepsis is essential
(*see* Principles of prevention of surgical sepsis, p. 4)
1. Mechanical cleansing
2. Debridement
3. Antisepsis (avoid alcohol)
4. Antitetanus measures
   a. Passive
   b. Active
5. Antibiotics
   a. Topical
   b. Systemic

Exploration needs
1. Avascular field (tourniquet)
2. Good light
3. Adequate anaesthesia
4. On table X-ray facilities
5. Wide exposure, converting laceration to a Z-incision
6. Preserve all viable skin and aim to get primary skin cover, either closing without tension or by skin graft

Nerve injury
1. Digital nerves
   Primary repair with epineural suture
2. Major nerves – indication to explore
   a. Open injury
   b. Closed injury with failure of recovery at expected rate of 100 mm in 100 days (follow with Tinnell's test)
   c. 90% of closed nerve injuries are neurapaxia but physical nerve damage must be suspected if there is no evidence of physiological recovery after 48–72 hours

Problem with major nerve repair
1. Arguments against primary repair
   a. Inexperience of surgeon
   b. Available facilities for microsurgery
   c. Epineurium is very thin for the first 2 weeks
   d. Higher incidence of anastomotic neuroma
   e. Nature of injury and size of defect
2. Therefore aim for initial skin cover and delayed repair; at 6 weeks there is good epineural tissue to suture and nerve viability can be more accurately assessed

Nerve repair
1. All nerve repairs should be performed after the tourniquet is released as an intraneural haematoma may jeopardise the repair
2. Examine fascicles using the operating microscope as their arrangements change every centimetre
3. Use 5/0 Prolene for epineural suture
4. Consider cable nerve graft for a large defect of less than 10 cm, using greater auricular nerve as a donor
5. Ulnar nerve length can be gained by anterior transposition at the elbow (*see* ulnar nerve transposition, p. 184)
6. Support in a cast for 2 weeks

Tendon repair
1. Mallet finger
   a. Resisted extension injury either tearing the tendon or avulsing the base of the distal phalanx at the insertion of the extensor tendon

b. 50% will recover after 4 weeks in a hypertension splint
2. Boutonniere
   a. Rupture of central slip of extensor tendon with subluxation of the interphalangeal joint
   b. Closed injury – early reduction with hyperextension splint
   c. Open injury – attempt repair

Flexor tendons of hand
Classical teaching – Burnell

Hand is divided into three zones

	Region	Management
Proximal	Proximal to metacarpophalangeal joint	Primary repair
Mid-zone	Between metacarpophalangeal joint and proximal interphalangeal	Delayed repair since tendons usually involved
Distal zone	Distal to proximal interphalangeal joint tendon	Primary repair of flexor digitorum profunda

(Experienced hand surgeons advocate primary repair for all three zones if both technically possible and the surgeon sufficiently experienced)
1. Always repair flexor tendons on their volar surface since they receive their blood supply by vincula which are usually on the palmar surface
2. Use non absorbable monofilament sutures

Postoperatively
1. Elevate the arm
2. Encourage early exercise and active splintage to reduce adhesions

Appendix

Operation planner for common operations

Operation	FBC	SMAC	CXR	ECG	Clotting	G&S/XM
Breast surgery						
Simple mastectomy	X	X	X	X	X	X
Radical mastectomy	X	X	X	X	X	X
Breast reconstruction	X	X	X	X	X	2
Cardiothoracic surgery						
Oesophageal dilatation	X	X	X	X	X	X
Oesophagectomy (all types)	X	X	X	X	X	4
Oesophageal transection (varices)	X	X	X	X	X	6
Oesophageal atresia surgery	X	X	X		X	2
Thoracotomy	X	X	X	X	X	2
Pulmonary lobectomy/ pneumonectomy	X	X	X	X	X	2
Coronary artery bypass graft	X	X	X	X	X	4
Cardiac valve replacement	X	X	X	X	X	4
Vascular surgery						
Femoral embolectomy	X	X	X	X	X	X
Femoropopliteal/distal bypass	X	X	X	X	X	X
Femoro/axillo-femoral bypass	X	X	X	X	X	X
Aortoiliac/bifemoral bypass	X	X	X	X	X	2
Elective repair of aortic aneurysm	X	X	X	X	X	4
Repair of ruptured aortic aneurysm	X	X	X	X	X	6
Carotid endarterectomy	X	X	X	X	X	X
Percutaneous angioplasty	X	X	X	X	X	X
Amputation of the leg	X	X	X	X	X	X

ABGs	X-ray	ITU	Bowel prep	Anti-biotics	Mark site	Comments
						Results of cytology, US and mammogram
						Results of cytology, US and mammogram
						Exclude local recurrence
						Barium swallow, oesophagoscopy and biopsies
X		X	X	X		Barium swallow, oesophagoscopy and biopsies
X		X	X	X		Neomycin and lactulose for encephalopathy
		X	X	X		
X	X	X		X		
X	X	X		X		Bronchoscopy and mediastinoscopy, biopsies
X		X		X		Coronary angiograms
X		X		X		Echocardiography and radiology
					X	Full anticoagulation if diagnosis suspected
				X	X	Angiography and Doppler ankle pressures
				X	X	Angiography and Doppler ankle pressures
		X		X		Angiography and Doppler ankle pressures
X		X		X		US/CT of aneurysm, Doppler ankle pressures
X		X		X		Resuscitate on way to theatre
X		X			X	Angiograms, Doppler studies
					X	Doppler angle pressure studies
X				X	X	

Operation	FBC	SMAC	CXR	ECG	Clotting	G&S/XM
Orthopaedic operations						
Operations for shoulder dislocation	X	X	X	X	X	X
Open reduction/fixation of arm fractures	X	X	X	X	X	
Amputations of the arm	X	X	X	X	X	
Surgery for fractured neck of fermur	X	X	X	X	X	X
Total hip replacement	X	X	X	X	X	2
Internal fixation of fractured femur	X	X	X	X	X	X
Total knee replacement	X	X	X	X	X	X
Open fixation of leg fractures	X	X	X	X	X	X
Arthroscopic procedures	X	X	X	X	X	
Laminectomy	X	X	X	X	X	X
Spinal fusion	X	X	X	X	X	4
Surgery for osteomyelitis	X	X	X	X	X	X
Head, neck and endocrine						
Block dissection of the neck	X	X	X	X	X	2
Parotidectomy	X	X	X	X	X	
Excision of branchial cyst	X	X	X	X	X	
Thyroidectomy	X	X	X	X	X	X
Parathyroidectomy	X	X	X	X	X	X
Excision of thyroglossal cyst	X	X	X	X	X	
Adrenalectomy	X	X	X	X	X	2
Tracheostomy	X	X	X	X	X	
Laryngectomy	X	X	X	X	X	4
Gastric operations						
Gastrostomy	X	X	X	X		
Vagotomy (all types)	X	X	X	X		
Pyloric stenosis (child)	X	X				X
Pyloric stenosis (adult)	X	X	X	X		X
Partial gastrectomy	X	X	X	X		2
Total gastrectomy	X	X	X	X	X	2
Thoracoabdominal gastrectomy	X	X	X	X	X	4
Heller's operation	X	X	X	X		X
Surgery for bleeding DU/GU	X	X	X	X	X	4
Repair of hiatus hemia	X	X	X	X		X

ABGs	X-ray	ITU	Bowel prep	Anti-biotics	Mark site	Comments
					X	
				X	X	Radiology, check peripheral pulses
					X	
X	X			X	X	Radiology
	?X			X	X	Radiology
				X	X	Radiology
				X	X	Radiology
	X			X	X	Radiology and check peripheral pulses
					X	Radiology
						Results of CT/MRI, document neurology
X	X	X		X		Radiology, document neurology
				X		Radiology, results of microbiology
				X	X	Results of cytology, EUA and biopsies
					X	Sialogram, US/CT, check 7th nerve
					X	Cytology and US
						US/thyroid scan, thyroid function, recurrent nerve
						Serum Ca^2, PTH, US/CT, check vocal cords
						US/thyroid scan
		?X			X	Adrenal function tests, US/CT, angiogram, MIBG
		X				
X		X		X		EUA and biopsy results
						Results of gastric secretion studies
X						Correct dehydration and acid-base imbalance
X				X		Correct dehydration and acid-base imbalance
				X		Barium radiology and biopsy results
X		?X		X		Barium radiology and biopsy results
X		X		X		Barium radiology and biopsy results
						Barium swallow and oesophageal manometry
X		?X		X		Results of preoperative endoscopy
						Results of radiology and endoscopy

Operation	FBC	SMAC	CXR	ECG	Clotting	G&S/XM	
Hepatobiliary operations							
Cholecystectomy (all types)	X	X	X	X	X	X	
Exploration of the CBD	X	X	X	X	X	X	
Choledochoduodenostomy	X	X	X	X	X	X	
Hepatic jejunostomy	X	X	X	X	X	4	
Hepatectomy (right/left)	X	X	X	X	X	6	
Pancreatoduodenectomy (Whipple)	X	X	X	X	X	4	
Distal pancreatectomy	X	X	X	X	X	2	
Splenectomy	X	X	X	X	X	platelets+2	
Shunt for portal hypertension	X	X	X	X	X	4	
Drainage of pseudocyst	X	X	X	X	X	2	
Small and large bowel							
Laparotomy for intestinal obstruction	X	X	X	X		2	X
Laparotomy for Crohn's disease	X	X	X	X	X	2	
Appendicectomy	X	X	X	X			
Right hemicolectomy	X	X	X	X		X	
Left hemicolectomy	X	X	X	X		X	
Sigmoid colectomy	X	X	X	X		X	
Hartmann procedure	X	X	X	X		X	
Subtotal colectomy	X	X	X	X		2	
Colectomy for fulminent colitis	X	X	X	X	X	4	
Anterior resection of the rectum	X	X	X	X		2	
Abdominoperineal resection of rectum	X	X	X	X		3	
Repair of rectal prolapse	X	X	X	X		X	
Urology (always send MSSU for MC&S)							
Endoscopic resection of bladder tumour	X	X	X	X	X	X	
TURP	X	X	X	X	X	X	
Simple nephrectomy	X	X	X	X	X	X	
Radical nephrectomy	X	X	X	X	X	3	
Pyelo- or uretero-lithotomy	X	X	X	X	X	X	

ABGs	X-ray	ITU	Bowel prep	Anti-biotics	Mark site	Comments
	X			X		US report
	X			X		Radiology and vitamin K
	X			X		Radiology and vitamin K
	X	?X		X		Radiology and vitamin K
X	?X	X		X		Results of CT and angiography
		X		X		CT, angiography and vitamin K
		?X		X		Results of CT
		?X		X		Pneumococcus vaccination
X		X		X		Oral neomycin and lactulose for encephalopathy
	?X			X		Results of US/CT
				X		Rehydrate and resuscitate
				X	X	Results of barium studies
				X		
			X	X		Results of barium studies/colonoscopy
			X	X		Results of barium studies/colonoscopy
			X	X		Results of barium studies/colonoscopy
			?X	X	X	Results of barium studies/colonoscopy
			X	X		Results of barium studies/colonoscopy
X		X		X	X	Rehydrate and resuscitate
			X	X		Results of barium studies/colonoscopy
			X	X	X	Results of barium studies/colonoscopy
			X	X		Results of rectal manometry
				X		IVU and urine cytology results
				X		Bladder US, urodynamics, PSA/acid phosphatase
				X	X	IVU/US
		?X		X	X	IVU/US/CT and angiogram
	X			X	X	X-ray on way to theatre, position of stone

Operation	FBC	SMAC	CXR	ECG	Clotting	G&S/XM
Urology (always send MSSU for MC&S) (Contd)						
Nephroureterectomy	X	X	X	X	X	2
Pyeloplasty	X	X	X	X	X	X
Partial cystectomy	X	X	X	X	X	X
Radical cystectomy	X	X	X	X	X	6
Urinary diversion (ileal conduit)	X	X	X	X	X	X
Ureteric reimplantation	X	X	X	X	X	X
Kidney transplantation	X	X	X	X	X	X
Repair of vesicovaginal/rectal fistula	X	X	X	X	X	2
Urethroplasty	X	X	X	X	X	X

G&S/XM is group and save or units cross matched; ABGs are arterial blood gases and respiratory function tests; ITU means book an ITU bed; X-ray means intra-operative radiology; radiology means results of previous X-rays.

ABGs	X-ray	ITU	Bowel prep	Anti-biotics	Mark site	Comments
				X	X	IVU/US urine cytology and cytoscopy
				X	X	IVU and renogram
				X		Cytoscopy, biopsies, rectal US, pelvic CT
		X	X	X	X	Cystoscopy, biopsies, rectal US, pelvic CT
			X	X	X	
				X		
X		X		X		Blood group and tissue type
			X	X		IVU and barium enema results
				X		Results of urethroscopy and urethrogram

Index